Endodontic Pain

Paul A. Rosenberg

Endodontic Pain

Diagnosis, Causes, Prevention and Treatment

Springer

Paul A. Rosenberg, DDS
Department of Endodontics
New York University College of Dentistry
New York, NY
USA

ISBN 978-3-642-54700-3 ISBN 978-3-642-54701-0 (eBook)
DOI 10.1007/978-3-642-54701-0
Springer Heidelberg New York Dordrecht London

Library of Congress Control Number: 2014940755

Printed on acid-free paper

Springer is part of Springer Science+Business Media (www.springer.com)

This book is dedicated to my wife, Maxine, whose encouragement and editorial assistance were essential to the completion of this book.

Foreword

The US Institute of Medicine has recently reported that more Americans experience chronic pain than the total number of patients experiencing cancer, heart disease, and diabetes combined. Thus, effective pain diagnosis and treatment are major challenges that impact all health-care providers. And yet, in many ways, pain is the lost stepchild of professional education. No "Department of Pain" exists. Instead, often a junior faculty member provides a survey course on anesthesia and analgesia, with additional lectures on diagnostic methods and evaluation strategies scattered among several other clinical disciplines. The result is a patchwork quilt of knowledge that too often is fragmentary, disjointed, and out of date. The present text by Professor Paul Rosenberg directly addresses this problem. Drawing upon his immense clinical expertise and leavened with an extensive knowledge of the latest research findings, Professor Rosenberg has created a tapestry for treating the pain patient that is comprehensive, unified, and up to date.

This text is organized in a logical fashion, and each chapter is presented in a similar fashion. Thus, the busy practitioner can quickly jump to a specific stand-alone chapter or can review related chapters. This feature allows one to efficiently consider specific details for individual patients. For example, do you have a patient with a post-endodontic "flare-up"? You can quickly jump to Chap. 7 and rapidly review diagnostic criteria, risk factors, and treatment strategies. Moreover, each chapter is filled with clinical tips which provide essential summaries of key points that can be successfully incorporated into practice. This is a gold mine of practical information designed for ease of use in a practice setting.

In addition, the entire book can serve as a class text. Although each chapter is written in a stand-alone fashion, there is minimal overlap between chapters. In addition, many chapters end with a self-assessment section often linked to a *patient narrative*. Again, the emphasis is a practical wisdom that directly services diagnosing and treating the pain patient. The overall text provides a solid text for an entire course in pain diagnosis and treatment.

Two additional features greatly enhance this text. First, the extensive use of clinical images and flow charts illustrates key concepts and greatly facilitates their incorporation into treatment. This is particularly important since a good picture truly is often worth a thousand words. Second, the accompanying DVD provides rapid access to this information including the opportunity for patient education using the associated clinical images.

In today's busy practice, it is difficult to find single, integrated sources of information that are designed for immediate application in diagnosing and treating the pain patient. This is a textbook that belongs not on your bookshelf but right on your desk. I am confident that it will increase your ability to efficiently manage these often complex clinical conditions.

Ken M. Hargreaves DDS, PhD
UT Health Science Center San Antonio
San Antonio, TX
USA

A Note to the Reader

In an effort to facilitate the use of this text, each chapter has been written as a stand-alone section. To a large extent, this will make it unnecessary for the reader to repeatedly move back and forth between chapters. However, there are some subjects which are introduced in one chapter and further developed in another. I hope that you will find this approach to be useful.

New York, NY, USA Paul A. Rosenberg, DDS

Acknowledgments

I want to thank the faculty of the Dr. Ignatius N. and Sally Quartararo Department of Endodontics at New York University College of Dentistry for their dedication to generations of students. I want to recognize Dr. Asgeir Sigurdsson for his continued support of this project. To the staff, Joseph Pellicciari, Nida Ahmed, Edna Afiriyie, and Eugene Podborits, I also extend my thanks for their support during the preparation of this manuscript.

I also want to acknowledge Dr. Paul Duncan Eleazer for and Dr. Matthew Malek for THEIR meticulous review of the manuscript his meticulous review of the manuscript. Dr. Kenneth Hargreaves has been a valued mentor and friend for many years. His research and scholarship, in the area of pain, have made a profound impact on patient care and have been extremely important to me in my efforts.

Contents

Diagnosis

1

1.1 Introduction

The International Association for the Study of Pain has defined pain as "an unpleasant sensory and emotional experience associated with actual or potential tissue damage or described in terms of such damage." This text will review both sensory and emotional aspects of pain and their relationship to endodontic practice.

At an initial consultation concerning pain, there are an incredible number of factors to be considered. Among them are biological, psychological, and psychosocial factors that have an influence on a patient's pain and their interaction with the dentist.

The diagnostic process requires organization of a mass of information drawn from a written medical history, a dialogue with the patient, radiographs, sensibility tests, and clinical examination. The diagnostic process proceeds in a logical, systematic manner leading to a synthesis of the findings. Quick judgments should be avoided until all of the data is collected.

This chapter will review varied aspects of the diagnostic process.

A good initial question to start a dialogue with the patient is "How can I help you?" Depending on the patient's personality and verbosity, this may lead to an extensive description of the patient's pain or a brief noncontributory response. Even at this early stage of the diagnostic process, listening closely can provide meaningful clues about the patient's pain and the direction to take the diagnostic process.

1.2 Medical History

The medical history is an important early step in the endodontic diagnostic process. It is advisable to use a written form supplemented by a conversation with the patient.

Often a patient may return a written form with little or no information provided. However, when asked if there is any additional information about past or present illnesses or medication, a stream of important medical details is presented.

P.A. Rosenberg, *Endodontic Pain*,
DOI 10.1007/978-3-642-54701-0_1, © Springer-Verlag Berlin Heidelberg 2014

A dialogue pertaining to the medical history could start with the following statement: "Is there anything in your medical history, past or present that has not been covered on the form?" Some patients are reluctant to provide portions of their medical history in writing but are willing to discuss it in privacy.

It must be determined if there are medical conditions or medications that could cause or affect the patient's symptoms or modify the diagnostic inquiry. Examples of medical conditions that may require consultation with the patient's physician, prior to treatment, include recent myocardial infarction, heart valve surgery, recent joint replacements, liver disease, and poorly controlled diabetics. The clinician is advised to have ready access, during the diagnostic and treatment planning process, to a text that can provide guidance in the treatment of medically compromised patients. A good example of such a text is *Little and Falace's Dental Management of the Medically Compromised Patient* [12]. Also important is ready access to physicians for consultation.

1.2.1 Diabetes

Patients taking insulin for diabetes must adhere to their diet. Consumption of adequate calories and medication at proper intervals is important to determine before treatment is initiated. Failing to eat in accordance with their diabetes management plan may result in a hypoglycemic event. A hypoglycemic reaction also may be due to an overdose of insulin or an oral hypoglycemic agent [12].

Pulps from patients with diabetes tend to have limited capillary exchange, collateral circulation, impaired immune response, increased risk of acquiring pulp infection (especially anaerobic ones), or necrosis, besides toothache and occasional tendency toward pulp necrosis caused by ischemia. In regard to molecular pathology, hyperglycemia is a stimulus for bone resumption, inhibiting osteoblastic differentiation and reducing bone recovery [11].

A study reviewed data from electronic patient records. It investigated the effect of diabetes mellitus on endodontic treatment outcome. It determined that patients with diabetes have increased periodontal disease with endodontic involvement compared with patients who did not have diabetes. There was also a trend toward increased symptomatic periradicular disease in patients with diabetes who received insulin, as well as flare-ups in all patients with diabetic disease [5].

Two years or longer postoperatively, 68 % of cases followed were successful. Older age, absence of preoperative lesions, presence of permanent restorations, and longer postoperative evaluation periods all were associated with a successful outcome. A multivariate analysis showed that in cases with preoperative periradicular lesions, history of diabetes was associated with a significantly reduced successful outcome. It was concluded that patients with diabetes have increased periodontal disease in teeth with endodontic problems and have reduced likelihood of success of endodontic treatment in cases with preoperative periradicular lesions [5].

Signs and Symptoms of Insulin Reaction

Mild Stage
- Hunger
- Weakness
- Tachycardia
- Pallor
- Sweating
- Paresthesia

Moderate Stage
- Incoherence
- Uncooperativeness
- Belligerence
- Lack of judgment
- Poor orientation

Severe Stage
- Unconsciousness
- Tonic or clonic movements
- Hypotension
- Hypothermia
- Rapid pulse

1.2.2 Liver Disease

Patients with liver disease and/or alcoholism require special consideration in terms of drugs to be used in conjunction with treatment. For example, a history of liver disease affects the choice of analgesics and precludes the use of acetaminophen.

Alcoholic patients with cirrhosis may require increased amounts of local anesthetics or additional anxiolytics due to liver enzyme induction and central nervous system effects of alcohol [12]. Dental drugs metabolized primarily by the liver include lidocaine (Xylocaine), mepivacaine (Carbocaine), prilocaine (Citanest), and bupivacaine (Marcaine). Their safety depends on the dose of the drug used and the severity of liver disease. Aspirin, acetaminophen (Tylenol), codeine, meperidine (Demerol), and ibuprofen (Motrin) should be avoided or used in a limited dose. Sedatives such as diazepam (Valium) and barbiturates should also be avoided or used in a limited amount depending on the severity of liver disease. The antibiotics metronidazole and vancomycin should also be avoided in the presence of severe liver disease (accute hepatitis and cirrhosis) [12].

Clinical Tips

- Prior to initiating treatment for patients with a history of liver disease, it is important for the clinician to review the relationship of drugs to be used (local anesthetics, analgesics, antibiotics, and sedatives) and their effect on the liver [12].
- When questions exist, consultation with the patient's/physician prior to treatment is always appropriate.

Drug and Alcohol Abuse

Abuse of drugs and alcohol is a growing public health worldwide problem. It impacts many areas of life including health care. Inevitably, dental practitioners will encounter patients whose desire for drugs seems inappropriate based on their actual therapeutic need. Dental/medical management of painful conditions and ascertaining the actual level of pain can be challenging especially in alcoholic patients or drug abusers.

1.2.3 Chronic Facial Pain

A history of chronic facial pain or headaches provides an important clue indicating that the clinician will have to differentiate between non-odontogenic and odontogenic pain.

There is recent evidence that a history of chronic painful conditions (e.g., temporomandibular dysfunction or chronic headaches) may predispose a patient to pain associated with endodontic treatment. A history of chronic painful conditions represents a potentially significant finding [16, 17].

1.3 History of the Chief Complaint

The patient's description of the onset of pain, its intensity, and what relieves it provides vital clues to the clinician. A key question for patients concerns the origin of their pain.

When a patient describes a "toothache," the clinician should not accept that as a final diagnosis. The description of a "toothache" must be verified through interpretation of the history and multiple sensibility and clinical tests and radiographs in order to be sure that the pain is actually odontogenic in nature.

Clinical Tips

- Absence of any specific dental complaint is a valuable clue indicating possible non-odontogenic origin of pain.

The history of the chief complaint is a starting point in differentiating odontogenic and non-odontogenic pain. Listening closely to the patient's dental history is a critical part of the diagnostic process. An astute diagnostician listens, like an inquisitive detective collecting information and synthesizing it. Actually, the collection of information starts at the moment the patient enters the treatment area.

The patient's personality is an important factor. Is the patient extremely anxious and non-communicative, or is the person calm and able to clearly describe their pain? How the patient responds during the diagnostic phase of treatment provides insight into their level of anxiety, and that is important as diagnosis and treatment progresses.

Often, the dentist can make a tentative diagnosis based on the information provided by the patient. One of the first considerations is to determine whether or not the symptoms indicate an odontogenic or non-odontogenic cause. That point represents a critical fork in the road for the clinician and patient. An important question, concerning odontogenic vs. non-odontogenic causation, includes a question concerning what provokes the pain. Others include: "How long have you had the pain?" "What words would you use to describe the pain?" "How long does it last?" "What stops the pain?"

1.3.1 Dental History

The dental history should also include details concerning past dental experiences including recent restorations and periodontal treatment. Either of those could cause postoperative symptoms that may complicate the diagnosis.

The history provides important insight into the patient's level of dental sophistication in terms of how they value preservation of their natural dentition. For example, a patient missing numerous teeth and having poor oral hygiene is an unlikely candidate for complex treatment with a questionable prognosis. Ultimately, the treatment plan must be individualized and appropriate for the patient. Prudent use of the patient's financial resources is another factor to consider.

Patients in severe pain may not be able to provide accurate information about the history of pain due to their physical and emotional distress. They may seem angry and depressed which are common outcomes of prolonged pain. Extreme pain can dominate a patient's life and cause a person's personality to totally change. Emily Dickinson, the American poet, expressed that feeling in a portion of a poem.

> PAIN has an element of blank;
> It cannot recollect
> When it began, or if there were
> A day when it was not.

It is not uncommon for a patient in acute pain at an emergency visit to seem angry and hostile, but after being relieved of pain the patient returns almost as a different human being. Understanding and empathy are important characteristics for a clinician treating a patient in pain.

Clinical Tips

- If the patient is a child, a parent or adult must be present to provide the medical/dental histories.
- If the patient is an adult with difficulty communicating, it is essential that another responsible person be present in order to translate and provide information concerning the medical/dental history.
- Serious complications may occur due to a language barrier resulting in an incomplete medical history. A specific example of this occurs when a patient or translator fails to communicate information concerning a history of a drug allergy. This error can lead to extremely serious complications.

1.3.2 Patient's Ability to Identify a Painful Tooth

A clinical study examined 79 endodontic emergency patients. Patients and dentists assessed the level of pain by using a verbal numeric rating scale (VNRS.) Results of that study indicated that patients presenting with odontogenic pain localized the painful tooth 73.3 % of the time. Patients experiencing periradicular pain localized the painful tooth (89 %) of the time, significantly more often than those without periradicular symptoms (30 %, $p<0.0001$.) It was concluded that the presence of periradicular pain increases the accuracy of pain localization. The VNRS is highly correlated with other pain scales and is an acceptable initial pain assessment tool for endodontic emergency patients [13].

Patients were frequently able to localize pain to the proper arch. The study found that the pain could be localized in 94.6 % of cases when there was pain to percussion and 90 % ($p=0.60$) for an overall arch localization of 92.3 %.

Clinical Tips

- It is advisable to think in terms of evaluating quadrants of teeth, using multiple tests, in both arches rather than testing only a suspect tooth.
- Always demonstrate the clinical tests in a normal quadrant before the suspect quadrant is evaluated.

1.3.3 Level of Pain

In assessing pain it is useful to have the patient describe the level of pain on a scale of 1–10. A written scale can be used for the patient to self-assess their level of pain. It is helpful in gauging the patient's progress or regression, if the patient must return for an additional diagnostic visit.

Some clinicians add descriptors to numbers such as "worst pain imaginable" for number 10 or "barely noticeable" for number 1 and ask the patient to indicate where they fall on that scale (Fig. 1.1).

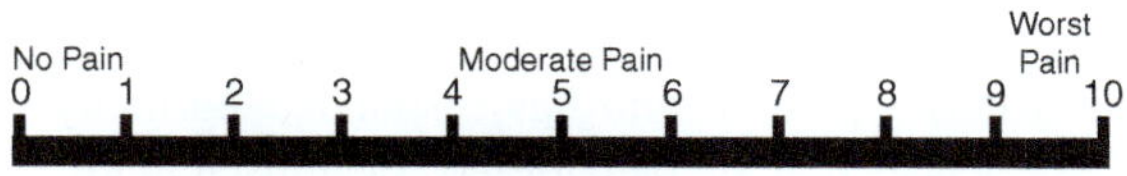

Fig. 1.1 Pain scale

1.4 What Provokes Pain?

It is important to determine what provokes the patient's pain and medications that provide relief. Understanding when the pain started also provides an important diagnostic clue. For example, pain that started years or months ago and remains at a low level does not fit the common profile of endodontic pain. Pulpal pain when initiated usually increases over a relatively short period of time. A vague response to the question of "What brings the pain on?" should raise doubts about odontogenic causation.

1.4.1 Non-odontogenic Toothache

Non-odontogenic "toothache" is a less common finding than odontogenic toothache. Differentiating odontogenic from non-odontogenic pain can be a challenging process. There are basic steps that can *differentiate the site of where pain is experienced from the actual source of pain*. Definitive treatment should never be initiated until the source of pain is clearly identified.

Clinical Tips

- An important clue is the *absence* of pain when the suspect tooth or quadrant is tested with cold, heat, percussion, and palpation. This clue points the inquiry toward a non-odontogenic cause of pain.

The finding of non-odontogenic pain is often confirmed by the patient's description of the onset of pain. If the description omits any of the most common causes of dental pain (e.g., thermal sensitivity or pain during mastication), it is another important clue pointing toward non-odontogenic causation. While the precise cause of pain at that stage remains unknown, it is clear that an endodontic dental cause is unlikely.

1.4.2 Non-odontogenic Toothache of Myofascial Origin

A myofascial source may be the cause of a toothache due to referred pain. Myofascial pain is often described as a deep, dull, aching pain that may be associated with referred pain to a tooth. Finger pressure and palpation of a specific myofascial trigger point may result in both muscle and tooth pain. Further tests are then required to identify the primary cause of pain. Palpation of musculature is an essential part of the diagnostic process and is discussed further in Chap. 2. It is not uncommon to find that a patient who has responded normally to sensibility and clinical tests experiences pain on palpation of the musculature.

1.4.3 Maxillary Sinusitis

Non-odontogenic toothache of sinus or nasal mucosal origin may be due to viral, bacterial, or allergic rhinitis and may be expressed as referred pain in the maxillae or maxillary teeth experienced by the patient as a toothache. Bacteria-induced sinusitis pain is often characterized as severe, throbbing pain with a sense of pressure [9].

After a tentative diagnosis of pain due to sinus involvement, it is prudent to refer the patient to a physician for confirmation of the diagnosis and treatment.

Clinical Tips

Findings associated with a diagnosis of pain due to sinusitis:

- An important diagnostic finding is that more than one tooth may be sensitive to thermal testing and percussion.
- Teeth test is vital in the suspect quadrant.
- Maxillary premolars and molars are most commonly affected by sinusitis.
- Discomfort may be bilateral.
- Typically, pain and pressure increase as the patient's head is lowered between their knees.
- Maxillary local anesthesia may provide partial relief of pain.
- Sinusitis may be associated with seasonal allergies or upper respiratory infections.
- An antihistamine may provide relief of pain if the cause is sinusitis.
- Reduction of pain after intranasal application of a 4 % lidocaine spray has been reported and is considered diagnostic [7].

1.5 Local Anesthesia as a Diagnostic Tool

Local anesthesia can be of great value during the diagnostic process. Anesthetizing a suspect tooth, with a block or infiltration injection, should eliminate pain if the cause of pain is odontogenic.

If pain persists despite symptoms indicating a successful anesthetic block, it is an indication that the cause is not likely to be a tooth in that quadrant. The next step would be to check the opposing quadrant or consider non-odontogenic pain.

In the maxillary arch an infiltration injection can be used to achieve anesthesia, but the clinician must recognize that teeth adjacent to the injection site may also be affected by the anesthetic. If the local anesthetic infiltration fails to eliminate "toothache," referred pain becomes a more likely diagnosis.

Patients experiencing severe pain or those having a long history of pain prior to the dental visit may have difficulty achieving complete dental anesthesia. Peripheral sensitization of nociceptors and/or central sensitization may be the cause of the problem.

Clinical Tips

- An incomplete response to a local anesthetic can lead to a diagnostic error.

Although the anesthetic test provides valuable information, false positives are possible. Results of the test must be integrated with other diagnostic data to reach a conclusion about the origin of pain. In maxillary teeth the local anesthetic test provides only an approximation of the origin of pain because multiple teeth may be anesthetized even when intra-ligamental or intraosseous injections are used [10, 18]. The importance of multiple tests and radiographs cannot be overemphasized.

Clinical Tips

- Spontaneous unprovoked pain may indicate either odontogenic or non-odontogenic pain.
- Patients should be asked, "Where do you feel pain? Is the pain inside or outside of your mouth?"
- An indication of *non-odontogenic* pain occurs when provocation (e.g., application of a cold stimuli or percussion) of the presumed site of pain (the tooth) does not increase the pain.
- An indication of *odontogenic pain occurs* when provocation of the presumed site of pain (the tooth) increases tooth pain.
- A patient may state that " massaging the jaw" or the area of the temporomandibular joint relieves pain. That would be typical of pain associated with the joint or musculature but is not typical of an endodontic problem.
- Identification and treatment of myofascial pain may require the assistance of a clinician with advanced training in that area.

1.6 "Red Flag Words"

The patient's use of specific words to describe their pain is meaningful. Following are words that provide important clues during the differentiation of odontogenic and non-odontogenic pain.

1.6.1 Words Commonly Used to Describe Odontogenic Pain

- Throbbing
- Pulsating
- Dull ache
- Pressure
- Sharp

1.6.2 Words Commonly Used to Describe Non-odontogenic Pain

- Burning
- Tingling
- Electric
- Searing
- Stabbing

1.7 Neuropathic Pain

The International Association for the Study of Pain has defined neuropathic pain as "initiated or caused by a primary lesion or dysfunction in the nervous system" [14]. Neuropathic pain has its etiology in neural tissue rather than in the structures that it innervates [22]. Some neuropathic pains present as episodic pain and some are more continuous. Toothache of neuropathic origin can present as either episodic or continuous pain.

Episodic neuropathic pain is characterized by sudden bursts of electric-like pain referred to as neuralgia. When this type of paroxysmal pain is felt in a tooth, it can pose a significant diagnostic challenge for the clinician.

Clinical Tips
- Trigeminal neuralgia is the most common episodic neuropathic pain felt in the teeth [8].

1.7.1 Characteristics of Odontogenic Pain

- A dental cause of pain may be apparent during examination, e.g., caries, fracture, and defective restoration.
- Significant radiographic findings include caries, extensive restorations, periapical lesions, and a calcified pulp chamber when others appear normal.
- Dental symptoms: thermal sensitivity and pain during mastication or following pressure against a tooth.
- Local anesthesia relieves pain.
- Unilateral pain.
- Localized pain [8].

1.7.2 Characteristics of Non-odontogenic Pain

- Absence of apparent etiologic dental cause on radiographs or clinical examination.
- Local anesthesia does not relieve pain.
- Lack of history of specific cause of pain.
- Pain that crosses the midline.
- Pain described as tingling, shooting, and burning.
- Pain not localized.
- Pain associated with headache.
- Palpation of joint or musculature causes pain.
- Pain associated with emotional stress.
- Presence of multiple teeth that have had endodontic treatment in the same quadrant [8].

Clinical Research Concerning Referred Pain

In a series of 230 cases with a diagnosis of temporomandibular dysfunction, 85.0 % demonstrated referred pain with palpation of muscles or trigger points and 11.6 % of these patients had pain referred to the teeth [23]. Molars most frequently received referred pain from muscle or trigger point palpation, and the masseter muscles were the most common source. Palpation of the musculature during an examination can provide meaningful information.

1.8 Dentinal Hypersensitivity

A patient may present with a chief complaint of a sharp pain provoked during tooth brushing or while eating sweets. The patient may also state that he/she can replicate the pain by rubbing a fingernail against a specific area of the tooth. The initial impression might be one of an endodontic problem, but closer examination may indicate that dentinal hypersensitivity may be the cause of the patient's pain. Typical clinical findings include a vital tooth, gingival recession exposing dentin, sensitivity to air, and pain associated with scraping an explorer against the exposed root.

There are two theories concerning the cause of the problem. One involves fluid movement through dentinal tubules resulting in the activation of nociceptors in the inner dentin and pulp [24].

In contrast, exposed dentin that is not sensitive most likely has dentinal tubules that are occluded. Substances that occlude dentinal tubules, in sensitive dentin, are used to eliminate or reduce sensitivity. A second hypothesis for dental hypersensitivity is that some substances may diffuse through the dentin and act directly on pulpal nerves. These hypotheses may occur independently or together [8].

A survey of dentists determined that a variety of therapies are used to treat dentinal hypersensitivity [1]. The most successful treatment was found to be fluoride application. Also widely used were glutaraldehyde/HEMA, bonding agents, potassium nitrates, and restorative treatments. The survey also determined that observation, advice regarding tooth brushing, diet, and laser therapy were the least successful.

Despite the therapy used some teeth remain extremely sensitive to provoking stimuli. In those cases, devitalization of the tooth is the treatment of last resort.

1.9 Diagnostic Quandary

There are some cases that pose a diagnostic problem that cannot be resolved at the initial visit. After completing the examination, doubt may still persist about the pain being of odontogenic or non-odontogenic origin. In other cases the pain may be clearly odontogenic, but identifying the problem tooth remains questionable. In those situations the dentist–patient dialogue might sound like this:

> "I do not have definitive evidence allowing me to pinpoint the source of your pain. While a mandibular molar seems to be the cause of the problem some doubt does exist. I have used a number of tests but there is still a question about the origin of your pain. If we proceed using the existing evidence, it involves the risk of treating the wrong tooth. I suggest that we wait until the picture clarifies. If necessary, I can provide analgesics for the next few days, monitor your status and then reevaluate."

The intent is to present the patient with a clear picture of the situation, provide reasonable options, and share responsibility for a critical decision. Not following this course leaves the dentist in a high-risk situation with sole responsibility for the diagnosis and treatment. This approach also prevents a combative relationship between the dentist and patient during a stressful phase of treatment.

Good doctor–patient communication is essential during the diagnostic process. The communication should be open, frank, and never defensive. Most patients are highly appreciative of a cautious and thoughtful approach to their care.

1.10 Treat or Refer

At an emergency or diagnostic visit, after the dentist determines that the patient's pain/swelling is due to an endodontic problem, the next decision is to determine if they will treat the patient or refer to a specialist.

The American Association of Endodontists (AAE) has developed guidelines for assessing endodontic case difficulty. The forms are available at http://www.aae.org/guidelines/.

The AAE Endodontic Case Difficulty Assessment Form enables a clinician to assign a level of difficulty to each case. The form describes characteristics of cases with minimal, moderate, and high degrees of difficulty. This form lists criteria that can be used to identify cases that should be referred to a specialist (Fig. 1.2).

AAE Endodontic Case Difficulty Assessment Form and Guidelines

PATIENT INFORMATION

Name________________________

Address________________________

City/State/Zip________________________

Phone________________________

DISPOSITION

Treat in Office: Yes ☐ No ☐

Refer Patient to:

____

Date:________________________

Guidelines for Using the AAE Endodontic Case Difficulty Assessment Form

The AAE designed the Endodontic Case Difficulty Assessment Form for use in endodontic curricula. The Assessment Form makes case selection more efficient, more consistent and easier to document. Dentists may also choose to use the Assessment Form to help with referral decision making and record keeping.

Conditions listed in this form should be considered potential risk factors that may complicate treatment and adversely affect the outcome. Levels of difficulty are sets of conditions that may not be controllable by the dentist. Risk factors can influence the ability to provide care at a consistently predictable level and impact the appropriate provision of care and quality assurance.

The Assessment Form enables a practitioner to assign a level of difficulty to a particular case.

LEVELS OF DIFFICULTY

MINIMAL DIFFICULTY — Preoperative condition indicates routine complexity (uncomplicated). These types of cases would exhibit only those factors listed in the MINIMAL DIFFICULTY category. Achieving a predictable treatment outcome should be attainable by a competent practitioner with limited experience.

MODERATE DIFFICULTY — Preoperative condition is complicated, exhibiting one or more patient or treatment factors listed in the MODERATE DIFFICULTY category. Achieving a predictable treatment outcome will be challenging for a competent, experienced practitioner.

HIGH DIFFICULTY — Preoperative condition is exceptionally complicated, exhibiting several factors listed in the MODERATE DIFFICULTY category or at least one in the HIGH DIFFICULTY category. Achieving a predictable treatment outcome will be challenging for even the most experienced practitioner with an extensive history of favorable outcomes.

Review your assessment of each case to determine the level of difficulty. If the level of difficulty exceeds your experience and comfort, you might consider referral to an endodontist.

The contribution of the Canadian Academy of Endodontics and others to the development of this form is gratefully acknowledged.

The AAE Endodontic Case Difficulty Assessment Form is designed to aid the practitioner in determining appropriate case disposition. The American Association of Endodontists neither expressly nor implicitly warrants any positive results associated with the use of this form. This form may be reproduced but may not be amended or altered in any way.

Fig. 1.2 AAE endodontic case difficulty assessment form

AAE Endodontic Case Difficulty Assessment Form

Criteria and Subcriteria	Minimal Difficulty	Moderate Difficulty	High Difficulty
A. PATIENT CONSIDERATIONS			
Medical history	☐ No medical problem (ASA Class 1*)	☐ One or more medical problems (ASA Class 2*)	☐ Complex medical history/serious illness/disability (ASA Classes 3-5*)
Anesthesia	☐ No history of anesthesia problems	☐ Vasoconstrictor intolerance	☐ Difficulty achieving anesthesia
Patient disposition	☐ Cooperative and compliant	☐ Anxious but cooperative	☐ Uncooperative
Ability to open mouth	☐ No limitation	☐ Slight limitation in opening	☐ Significant limitation in opening
Gag reflex	☐ None	☐ Gags occasionally with radiographs/treatment	☐ Extreme gag reflex which has compromised past dental care
Emergency condition	☐ Minimum pain or swelling	☐ Moderate pain or swelling	☐ Severe pain or swelling
B. DIAGNOSTIC AND TREATMENT CONSIDERATIONS			
Diagnosis	☐ Signs and symptoms consistent with recognized pulpal and periapical conditions	☐ Extensive differential diagnosis of usual signs and symptoms required	☐ Confusing and complex signs and symptoms: difficult diagnosis ☐ History of chronic oral/facial pain
Radiographic difficulties	☐ Minimal difficulty obtaining/interpreting radiographs	☐ Moderate difficulty obtaining/interpreting radiographs (e.g., high floor of mouth, narrow or low palatal vault, presence of tori)	☐ Extreme difficulty obtaining/interpreting radiographs (e.g., superimposed anatomical structures)
Position in the arch	☐ Anterior/premolar ☐ Slight inclination (<10°) ☐ Slight rotation (<10°)	☐ 1st molar ☐ Moderate inclination (10-30°) ☐ Moderate rotation (10-30°)	☐ 2nd or 3rd molar ☐ Extreme inclination (>30°) ☐ Extreme rotation (>30°)
Tooth isolation	☐ Routine rubber dam placement	☐ Simple pretreatment modification required for rubber dam isolation	☐ Extensive pretreatment modification required for rubber dam isolation
Morphologic aberrations of crown	☐ Normal original crown morphology	☐ Full coverage restoration ☐ Porcelain restoration ☐ Bridge abutment ☐ Moderate deviation from normal tooth/root form (e.g., taurodontism, microdens) ☐ Teeth with extensive coronal destruction	☐ Restoration does not reflect original anatomy/alignment ☐ Significant deviation from normal tooth/root form (e.g., fusion, dens in dente)
Canal and root morphology	☐ Slight or no curvature (<10°) ☐ Closed apex (<1 mm in diameter)	☐ Moderate curvature (10-30°) ☐ Crown axis differs moderately from root axis. Apical opening 1-1.5 mm in diameter	☐ Extreme curvature (>30°) or S-shaped curve ☐ Mandibular premolar or anterior with 2 roots ☐ Maxillary premolar with 3 roots ☐ Canal divides in the middle or apical third ☐ Very long tooth (>25 mm) ☐ Open apex (>1.5 mm in diameter)
Radiographic appearance of canal(s)	☐ Canal(s) visible and not reduced in size	☐ Canal(s) and chamber visible but reduced in size ☐ Pulp stones	☐ Indistinct canal path ☐ Canal(s) not visible
Resorption	☐ No resorption evident	☐ Minimal apical resorption	☐ Extensive apical resorption ☐ Internal resorption ☐ External resorption
C. ADDITIONAL CONSIDERATIONS			
Trauma history	☐ Uncomplicated crown fracture of mature or immature teeth	☐ Complicated crown fracture of mature teeth ☐ Subluxation	☐ Complicated crown fracture of immature teeth ☐ Horizontal root fracture ☐ Alveolar fracture ☐ Intrusive, extrusive or lateral luxation ☐ Avulsion
Endodontic treatment history	☐ No previous treatment	☐ Previous access without complications	☐ Previous access with complications (e.g., perforation, non-negotiated canal, ledge, separated instrument) ☐ Previous surgical or nonsurgical endodontic treatment completed
Periodontal-endodontic condition	☐ None or mild periodontal disease	☐ Concurrent moderate periodontal disease	☐ Concurrent severe periodontal disease ☐ Cracked teeth with periodontal complications ☐ Combined endodontic/periodontic lesion ☐ Root amputation prior to endodontic treatment

*American Society of Anesthesiologists (ASA) Classification System

Class 1: No systemic illness. Patient healthy.
Class 2: Patient with mild degree of systemic illness, but without functional restrictions, e.g., well-controlled hypertension.
Class 3: Patient with severe degree of systemic illness which limits activities, but does not immobilize the patient.
Class 4: Patient with severe systemic illness that immobilizes and is sometimes life threatening.
Class 5: Patient will not survive more than 24 hours whether or not surgical intervention takes place.

www.asahq.org/clinical/physicalstatus.htm

Fig. 1.2 (continued)

1.11 "When Will the Pain Get Worse?"

Pain is the result of variables including host defense mechanisms, bacterial virulence factors, patient's level of anxiety, and the inflammatory/immune response. It is common for patients to have tolerable levels of pain for weeks or months prior to an acute exacerbation. Patients may comment "I can tolerate the current pain but how long do I have before it gets worse?" This is an impossible question to answer because of the unpredictable dynamic balance between irritants and host reaction.

Flare-ups are disturbing for patients and clinicians. It is not easy to explain to a patient why a tooth that was essentially painless before treatment became painful following treatment. To avoid that scenario, before a flare-up occurs, it is wise to discuss the possibility of pain and swelling. At that time emergency contact numbers and other similar information should be provided. This is usually reassuring to the patient and addresses a source of anxiety.

1.12 Patients' Descriptions of Symptoms

Patient's description of the history, onset, and intensity of their pain may not be dependable. Anxiety and fear interfere with patients' memory and accurate description of their symptoms. For example, a patient asked about a history of trauma may not recall a seemingly meaningless traumatic event that occurred years ago. A highly anxious patient may also not recall all of their medical history including medications they are taking and may not remember instructions given to them by the dentist. Anxiety may affect every level of treatment from diagnosis through intraoperative procedures.

1.12.1 Light Source and Visual Enhancement

A good light source and visual enhancement in the form of loupes or microscopy is important during the patient's examination. We cannot diagnose nor treat what we cannot see. The result of improving available light and magnification is usually dramatic and highly satisfactory for the clinician and the endodontic outcome.

The intraoral soft tissue examination starts with visual examination and palpation of the mucous membranes, gingiva, tongue, and floor of the mouth. The clinician should be looking for abnormalities of the mucous membranes including stomas, swellings, ulcerations, or precancerous lesions or cancerous lesions. A periodontal probe may be required when a significant periodontal defect is observed on

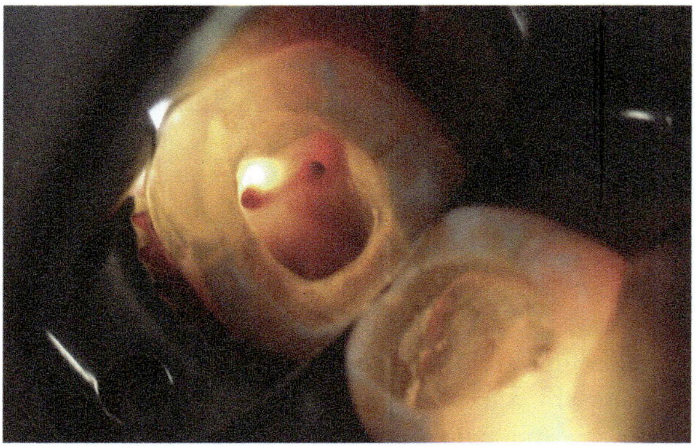

Fig. 1.3 Image of a molar chamber viewed through a surgical operating microscope

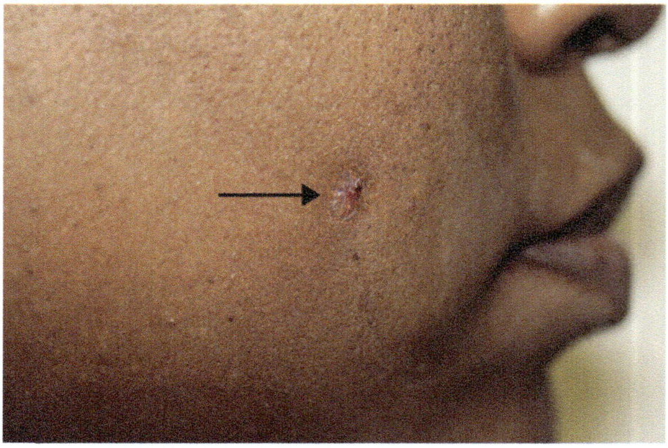

Fig. 1.4 *Arrow* points to an external stoma due to maxillary molar endodontic pathosis

radiographs or during visual examination. Both dorsal and ventral sides of the tongue and floor of the mouth should be examined using a gauze square to elevate the tongue.

Swellings should be gently palpated to determine their extent and if they are hard or fluctuant. This information will be important in determining the course of treatment at the visit. There is some disagreement among clinicians about whether or not to incise and drain only fluctuant swellings or hard swellings as well [3, 4] (Fig. 1.3).

1.12.2 Extraoral

The clinical examination starts with an extraoral examination. The clinician should look for signs of facial asymmetry that could be due to intraoral swelling. The clinician should palpate the joint area and evaluate tenderness. The lymph nodes should also be palpated while looking for signs of enlargement or sensitivity. Some skin lesions might seem to be dermatologic in nature but actually represent extraoral stomas signaling intraoral infection (Fig. 1.4).

If the patient experiences pain in the temporomandibular area while opening the mouth, that should lead to palpation of the musculature and a different path of inquiry that will differentiate muscle pain from pulp pain.

Patients with dental injuries may have concomitant head and neck injuries that are initially masked due to dental pain. During an examination, following a traumatic incident, the patient should be asked to move their head vertically and laterally to ensure normal movement. The eyes should be focused and move normally. Speech should also be normal without slurring. A significant number of seemingly dentoalveolar injuries have a head and neck component requiring a medical intervention. When in doubt it is never a mistake to secure a medical consultation.

Clinical Tips

- The results of sensibility tests in the weeks following a traumatic incident are suspect. They often produce false-negative or false-positive findings.
- Traumatized immature teeth, especially those with open apices, often do not provide accurate responses to sensibility tests.
- The sensibility tests do have value in providing an initial baseline, which can be compared to results of subsequent tests. It is essential that multiple tests be used to evaluate the status of the pulp.

1.12.3 Intraoral Examination

The intraoral examination should start with the buccal mucosa, floor of the mouth, throat, and gingiva. An oral cancer examination is part of this process. Visual examination and palpation are necessary to identify abnormalities, and a good light source is essential.

A thorough examination of the soft tissues may resolve a diagnostic puzzle. Unsuspected periodontal defects including food impaction areas can cause pain that mimics pulpal pain. Often the descriptive words used by a patient are the same for pulp or periodontal pain. The description can include words like "pressure, throbbing, tender to touch." A periodontal probe is useful in examining suspect areas and identifying stomas. An attempt should be made to trace all stomas to their source.

Clinical Tips

- An oral cancer screening should be part of every examination.
- The intraoral examination includes visual examination and palpation of the soft tissues including the tongue, sublingual tissue, throat, and gingiva.

1.12.4 Stomas: Biological Significance

A stoma represents a point of egress for drainage due to infectious/inflammatory conditions. The clinician is advised to attempt to trace the source of all stomas. Drainage follows the path of least resistance, and the results of tracing a tract can be surprising. It may indicate that the source of the tract is not the tooth initially suspected. Pulp sensibility testing of teeth in the quadrant would be the next logical step. Patients with stomas do not usually have pain. Continuing drainage represents decompression of the apical tissues, and the typical buildup of pressure causing pain does not occur in patients with a stoma.

Location of the stoma in the mucobuccal fold is significant. Stomas located in the gingival third are typically associated with a periodontal defect, while those in the middle third may be due to a fracture or perforation. A stoma in the apical third is more typical of an endodontic lesion.

Clinical Tips

- A patient should not be given an antibiotic to treat a stoma.
- While the stoma may appear to heal following the use of an antibiotic, it will return after the antibiotic is terminated because the medication is not delivered to a necrotic pulp, devoid of circulation, and does not address the basic microbiologic intra-canal source of the problem.
- Intra-canal microbes are the cause of the endodontic pathologic process, and they can only be eliminated by cleaning/shaping and irrigation.

Tracing a Sinus Tract

Use of a thin gutta-percha cone is recommended for tracing a sinus tract.

Using an orthodontic wire for tracing a stoma is not advisable. Due to its sharpness and rigidity, it may dissect through soft tissue creating its own pathway thus providing misleading diagnostic results.

An extraoral stoma can result from long-standing necrotic teeth with periapical lesions. Mandibular incisors and maxillary teeth may be associated with extraoral stomas. Extraoral stomas may be confused with a dermatologic lesion, and patients may present a history of extensive dermatologic treatment prior to a dental referral (Figs. 1.5, 1.6 and 1.7).

Clinical Tips

- Intraoral and extraoral stomas typically close during or immediately following successful endodontic treatment.
- When a stoma persists after treatment, it is possible that a missed canal or erroneous diagnosis may have occurred. The dentist should consider a concomitant periodontal lesion, root fracture, or undiscovered canal as the cause of the problem.

1.12.5 Endodontic–Periodontal Complications

Combined endodontic and periodontal pathosis may complicate the diagnostic process. The question often involves determining the primary cause of the patient's pain and or swelling. Several factors are important to note. If the tooth in question tests vital, it is an important indication that the primary cause of the problem is probably not endodontic. A non-vital response tends to indicate

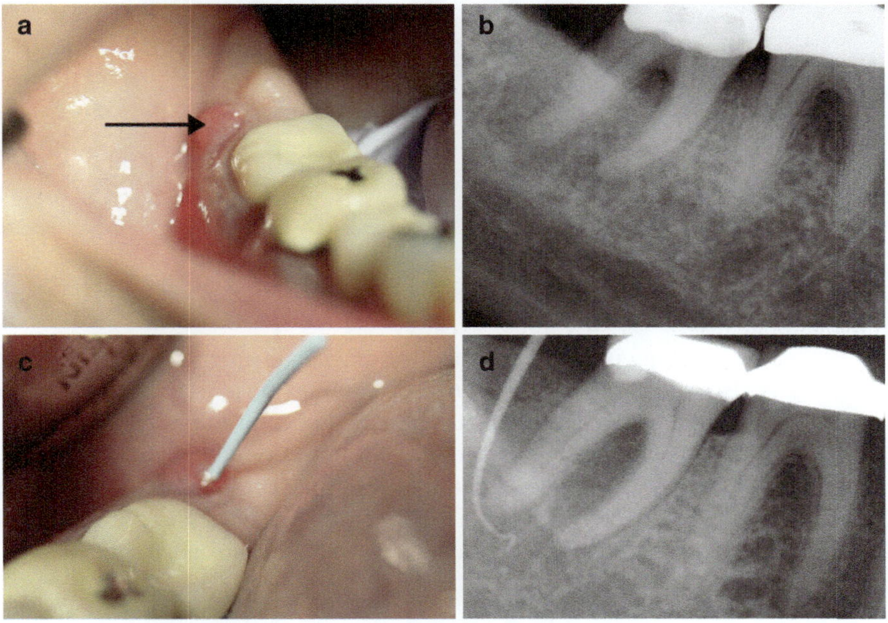

Fig. 1.5 (**a**) *Arrow* points to stoma distal to mandibular second molar. (**b**) Radiograph of mandibular second molar indicating periapical radiolucency associated with mesial and distal roots. (**c**) Gutta-percha cone inserted in stoma. (**d**) Radiograph of gutta-percha tracing sinus tract

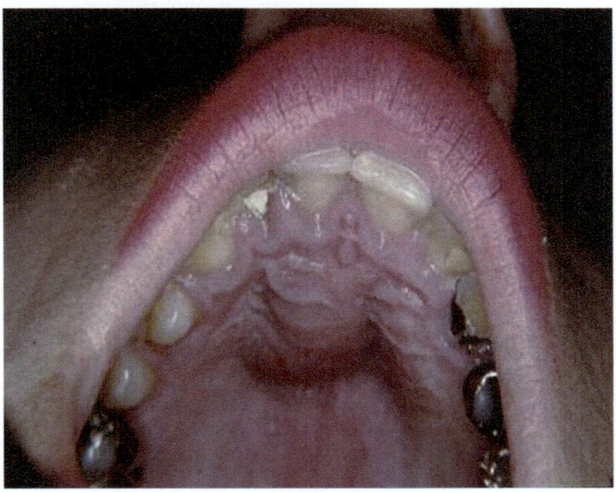

Fig 1.6 Palatal swelling associated with necrotic maxillary lateral incisor

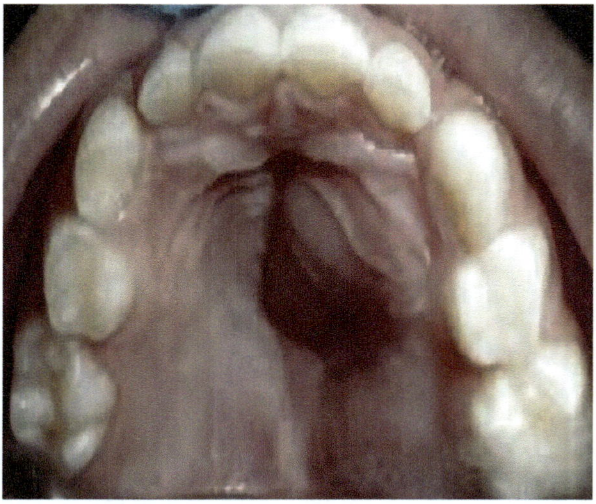

Fig. 1.7 Palatal swelling. Biopsy determined lesion was a rhabdomyosarcoma

periodontal causation, especially if there is a deep periodontal pocket and/or significant bone loss.

Periodontal probing is a critical part of the diagnostic process. Location of the swelling is also of diagnostic importance. A swelling close to the gingival margin in combination with a deep pocket is another indicator of periodontal causation. Often patients will present a history of chronic periodontal problems in the area being examined. In contrast endodontic swellings are typically found in the apical third of the mucobuccal fold. There are some instances where combined periodontal–endodontic lesions require both periodontal and endodontic therapy.

Clinical Tips

- Palpation is also an important part of the diagnostic process in endodontic–periodontal cases.
- Pain on palpation in the gingival or middle third of the mucobuccal fold, and an absence of pain in the apical third, should raise suspicions about a periodontal cause.
- Pain in the apical third of the mucobuccal fold is consistent with an endodontic problem, while pain in the gingival third is more typical of periodontal causation.

1.12.6 Treatment Planning

Treatment planning cases with endodontic/periodontal complications are complex. Among the factors involved is the patient's dental history. Does the patient have a strong desire to preserve his/her dentition, or is there evidence of neglect? Is there an economic factor involved? What is the prognosis for the proposed treatment?

In some situations an endodontist and/or a periodontist may provide valuable assistance as part of a team approach.

Clinical Tips

- The decision concerning whether to provide endodontic or periodontal therapy first or together is complex and best decided initially by directing therapy at the patient's symptoms.
- If the patient's chief complaint seems to be endodontic in origin, then endodontic treatment should be initiated.
- If the symptoms seem to stem from a periodontal defect, initial therapy should be directed at that problem.

1.12.7 Hard Tissue Examination

The hard tissue examination includes the palate and teeth. A good light source is invaluable in examining the palate for swellings or stomas that might otherwise be

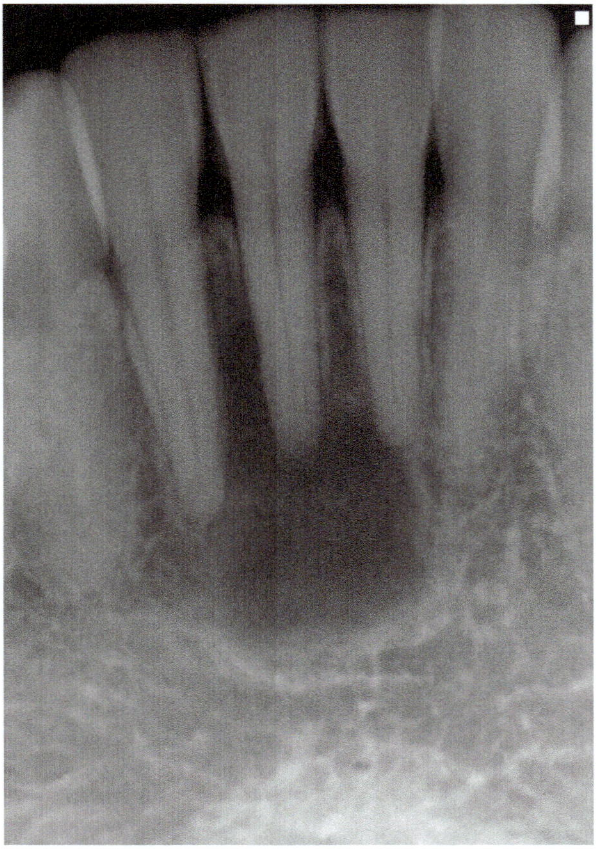

Fig. 1.8 Preoperative periapical lesion in the mandibular anterior region. All teeth tested vital. There was no history of trauma (Courtesy of Dr. Matthew Malek)

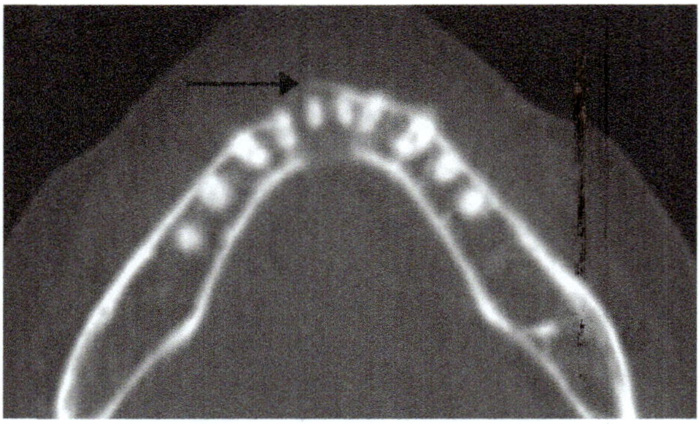

Fig. 1.9 Cone beam radiograph indicating labial and lingual breakdown of the bone; *arrow* points to labial bone breakdown

missed. The examination should be visual and also include palpation. Some suspect lesions may require biopsy to reach a diagnosis. Referral is often required in these cases (Figs. 1.8 and 1.9).

1.12.8 Teeth

The teeth are the last area for examination. Again, a good light source and visual enhancement are essential. The clinician should be examining large restorations for defects, potential cracks, and caries, all of which can be the cause of pulp pathosis.

Clinical Tips

- The root end of a maxillary lateral incisor is often curved to the disto-palatal. This can cause a swelling associated with the tooth to appear on the palate.
- Swellings, regardless of the location, may not be of endodontic origin. Definitive diagnosis of some lesions will require biopsy.

Biopsy

In some cases, final diagnosis is dependent upon biopsy results. Biopsy remains the gold standard of definitive diagnosis of questionable lesions. In endodontics, a classic indication for biopsy is a periapical lesion on radiograph associated with a tooth or teeth that test vital to sensibility tests.

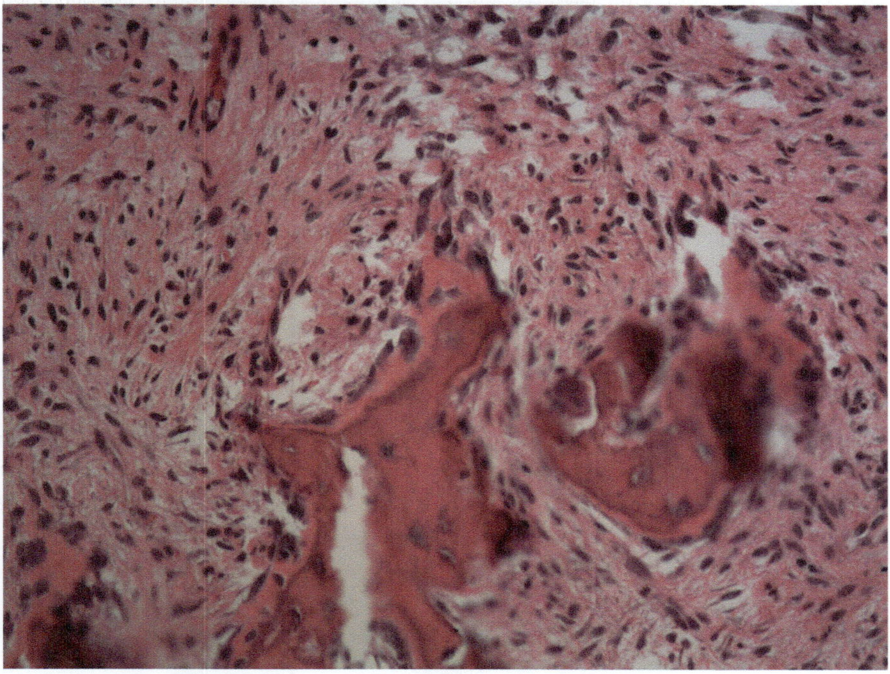

Fig. 1.10 Biopsy (H+E stain) indicating periapical cemento-osseous dysplasia (PCOD)

Neither panoramic nor cone beam radiographs (CBCT) can provide a definitive diagnosis of such lesions. A study compared the accuracy of CBCT compared to biopsy of endodontic surgical specimens. It was determined that biopsy remains the most valid diagnostic method in determining the cause of apical pathosis [20].

Cases requiring biopsy will often be referred to oral surgeons who are experienced at that procedure.

1.13 Complex Diagnostic Cases

In some complex cases, diagnosis of a periapical radiolucent lesion will require clinical and radiographic examinations, sensibility tests, CBCT, and biopsy. The following case report describes how various tests can be used in a logical, sequential manner in order to reach an evidence-based diagnosis.

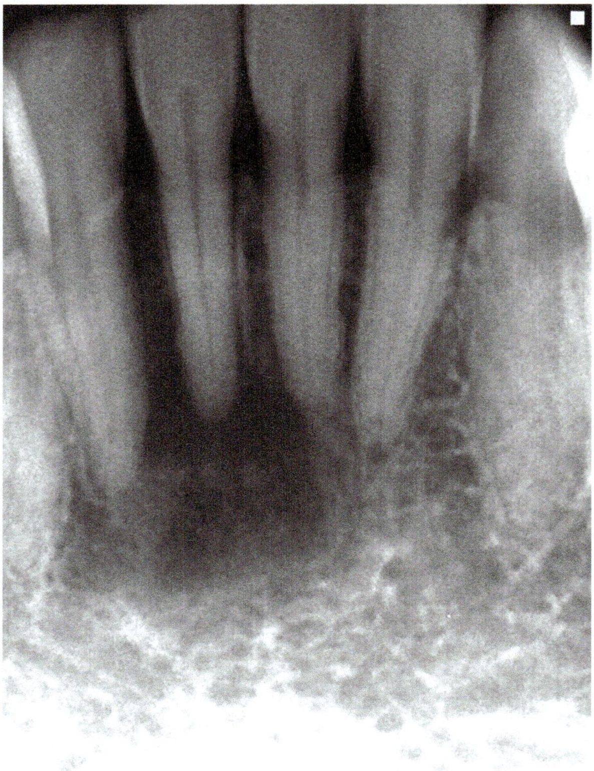

Fig. 1.11 The patient returned for evaluation after 1 year. No treatment was provided. There were no symptoms. One-year review radiograph

1.13.1 Case Report

The patient was a 59-year-old Hispanic female with a chief complaint of a small tender poorly defined, swelling of 1 week duration. Clinically, the swelling appeared deep in the mucobuccal fold and seemed to be associated with the apices of the mandibular right central and lateral incisors. It was tender to palpation and not fluctuant.

On periapical radiographs the lesion seemed to be associated with the apices of the mandibular right central and lateral incisors. All teeth in the area tested vital to cold and electricity.

The dental history did not indicate previous traumatic incidents or other notable events other than occasional, temporary swelling in the area. There was no significant medical history. Cone beam computed tomography (CBCT) revealed bony expansion (1 cm by 1 cm) associated with the suspect teeth and labial and lingual bony defects. A biopsy of the lesion followed in order to reach a definitive diagnosis (Figs. 1.10 and 1.11).

Differential diagnosis included non-endodontic unilocular radiolucent lesions that may possibly be found in the anterior mandibular region.

The differential diagnosis prior to biopsy included a wide range of possibilities. They included:

- Periapical cemento-dysplasia
- Central giant cell granuloma
- Cystic ameloblastoma
- Simple bone cyst (traumatic bone cyst)
- Central ossifying fibroma

Systemic diseases were also considered. They included:

- Renal osteodystrophy (this may cause radiolucent areas in the anterior mandible)
- Metastatic carcinoma
- Sarcoma

Biopsy findings were consistent with periapical cemento-osseous dysplasia (PCOD). The endodontist and oral surgeon and pathologist agreed that the case would be observed periodically, but there would be no treatment at that time. A 1-year review indicated no significant change in the lesion and no tenderness in the fold.

The clinical appearance of PCOD varies from being non-expansile and asymptomatic to being expansile and symptomatic. In complex diagnostic cases, a full range of diagnostic tools, radiographs, and a biopsy may be necessary to confirm a diagnosis.

1.14 Scheduling Considerations

If a vital case is to be treated using a multi-visit approach, it is suggested that the clinician allow 5 to 7 days between canal instrumentation and obturation in order to allow periradicular tissues to recover. By scheduling in this manner, the clinician and patient may often save time. If the patient presents several days after instrumentation (especially in vital teeth) with tenderness, then obturation is ill advised and often results in serious postoperative pain. By allowing time for recovery, following instrumentation, obturation is likely to result in a smooth postoperative course. When a case is to be treated in a single visit, adequate time must be scheduled so that the clinician can comfortably complete the procedure and not compromise the end result [19].

Clinical Tips

- Since profound inferior alveolar nerve block anesthesia may require 10–15 min or more, it is wise to consider that when scheduling a patient's appointment.

Appointments to fill non-vital cases should also be scheduled approximately 1 week after instrumentation in order to maximize the antimicrobial effect of the intra-canal dressing when calcium hydroxide is used and allow periapical tissues to recover from treatment procedures [6, 15].

However, patients with acute pain and/or swelling in non-vital cases should be seen every 24–48 h in order to monitor the patient's progress and bring the acute symptoms under control. In cases with persistent pain/swelling, frequent cleaning/shaping and irrigation with sodium hypochlorite is an important step in reducing the intra-canal bacterial flora. Long delays between visits contribute to the development of resistant microbial strains and should be avoided.

1.14.1 Single vs. Multiple Visits

Significant controversy exists over the question of whether it is preferable to complete endodontic therapy in single or multiple visits. Factors to be considered in the treatment plan include operator ability and experience; tooth conditions, e.g., vital or non-vital tooth; retreatment cases; symptomatic or asymptomatic cases; presence or absence of swelling; adequate treatment time; medical history and patient attitude; as well as anatomic and biological considerations.

A systematic review of randomized controlled clinical trials was conducted in order to provide evidence-based data to support dental decision making [2, 21]. The purpose of the systematic review was to investigate whether the effectiveness and frequency of short-term and long-term complications are different when an endodontic case is completed in one or multiple visits. It also investigated whether completion of root canal therapy in a single visit or during multiple visits makes any detectable difference in terms of clinical and radiologic success and in terms of both short-term and long-term complications.

No detectable difference was found in the effectiveness of root canal treatment in terms of radiologic success between single and multiple visits. Neither single-visit root canal treatment nor multiple-visit root canal treatment can prevent 100 % of short-term and long-term complications.

A systematic review and meta-analysis examined the best available evidence and determined that the difference in healing rate between single- and multiple-visit endodontic treatments of teeth with apical periodontitis was not statistically significant [2].

Clinical Tips

- The decision concerning the appropriate number of visits should be made on a case-by-case basis after considering the complexity of the case and biological factors including presence of a draining stoma or ongoing swelling.

Variables Considered in Endodontic Treatment Planning

- Is the patient symptomatic in terms of acute pain and/or swelling?
- Is there a stoma present?
- Is the tooth anatomically complex?
- Is there a full coverage or an extensive restoration present?
- If the patient is relatively asymptomatic, is it appropriate to complete the case in a single visit?
- Can the tooth be restored?
- Is there a periodontal component to the case?
- Is the patient's systemic health a factor?
- Will the dentist's skills allow treatment goals to be accomplished in a single visit?
- Is there sufficient time to complete the procedure without rushing?

1.15 Self-Assessment

1.15.1 Narrative 1

A 42-year-old female patient presents with a chief complaint of low-level, intermittent pain, of 6 months duration. She states that she can isolate the pain to the mandibular right first molar. There is no significant medical history. Her dental history includes numerous composite restorations, and she has good oral hygiene and no serious periodontal disease. The mandibular right first molar has a class 2 composite restoration of moderate depth. She is able to masticate without difficulty. A previous extraction of the maxillary right first molar occurred 2 years ago due to failed root canal treatment. The root canal therapy on that tooth was done in an attempt to alleviate pain in that area. Despite the extraction the patient describes continuing pain in that area as well as the opposing mandibular tooth. She describes the current pain as intense burning that starts in her tooth but then causes a severe headache. When asked what provokes the pain, the patient responds that it occurs spontaneously.

Clues

- The absence of any specific dental complaints is important.
- There is no mention of pain associated with mastication.

- The description of the pain as "intense burning" is not consistent with endodontic pain.
- The patient's prior history of an extraction following failed root canal treatment and continuing pain points toward non-dental causation.

Clinical Approach
- Periapical and bitewing radiographs must be reviewed.
- This should be followed by clinical and sensibility tests in the mandibular and maxillary quadrants.

What Would You Do?
There is probably a non-odontogenic cause of pain.
In the absence of any significant dental findings, the patient should be referred for consultation to a neurologist or facial pain specialist.

1.15.2 Narrative 2

The patient is a 36-year-old man in good health with a chief complaint of intermittent severe pain that started suddenly 3 days ago following dinner. He has excellent oral hygiene and numerous satisfactory dental restorations. The patient points to posterior teeth on the left side of the mandible while describing the pain. Pain is provoked by finger pressure against the left mandibular first molar. It has a deep composite restoration. There are no significant extra- or intraoral findings.

Clues
- Sudden onset of severe pain following mastication
- Acute sensitivity to pressure

Clinical Approach
- Periapical and bitewing radiographs should be reviewed.
- Clinical and sensibility tests in the left mandibular and maxillary quadrants.
- Transillumination with a fiber optic light source is a useful test in this situation to determine the presence of a fracture.
- Staining with methylene blue may indicate fracture line.
- A wooden bite block or Tooth Sleuth® (Professional Results Inc. Laguna, California) can be used to evaluate the possibility of a fracture. A sharp pain on closure or release of the bite is a symptom confirming fracture.
- A cone beam radiograph may reveal a fracture.

What Is Your Conclusion?
Probable fracture.
If fracture cannot be identified, endodontic access should be initiated. If pain is not relieved following endodontic instrumentation, it is likely that a fracture is the cause of the problem.

References

1. Cunha-Cruz J, Wataha JC, Zhou L et al (2010) Treating dentin hypersensitivity: therapeutic choices made by dentists of the northwest PRECEDENT network. J Am Dent Assoc 141(9): 1097–1105
2. Figini L, Lodi G, Gorni F et al (2008) Single versus multiple visits for endodontic treatment of permanent teeth: a Cochrane systematic review. J Endod 34(9):1041–1047
3. Flynn TR, Shanti RM, Hayes C (2006) Severe odontogenic infections, part 2: prospective outcomes study. J Oral Maxillofac Surg 64(7):1104–1113
4. Flynn TR, Shanti RM, Levi MH et al (2006) Severe odontogenic infections, part 1: prospective report. J Oral Maxillofac Surg 64(7):1093–1103
5. Fouad AF, Burleson J (2003) The effect of diabetes mellitus on endodontic treatment outcome: data from an electronic patient record. J Am Dent Assoc 134(1):43–51; quiz 117–118
6. Genet JM, Hart AA, Wesselink PR et al (1987) Preoperative and operative factors associated with pain after the first endodontic visit. Int Endod J 20(2):53–64
7. Graff-Radford SB (1991) Headache problems that can present as toothache. Dent Clin North Am 35(1):155–170
8. Hargreaves KM, Cohen S, Berman LH (2011) Cohen's pathways of the pulp. Mosby Elsevier, St. Louis
9. Hargreaves KM, Goodis HE (2012) Seltzer and Bender's dental pulp. Quintessence, Chicago
10. Kim S (1986) Ligamental injection: a physiological explanation of its efficacy. J Endod 12(10):486–491
11. Lima SM, Grisi DC, Kogawa EM et al (2013) Diabetes mellitus and inflammatory pulpal and periapical disease: a review. Int Endod J 46(8):700–709
12. Little JW, Falace DA, Miller C et al (2012) Dental management of the medically compromised patient. Mosby, St. Louis
13. McCarthy PJ, McClanahan S, Hodges J et al (2010) Frequency of localization of the painful tooth by patients presenting for an endodontic emergency. J Endod 36(5):801–805
14. Merskey H (2002) Clarifying definition of neuropathic pain. Pain 96(3):408–409
15. Mor C, Rotstein I, Friedman S (1992) Incidence of interappointment emergency associated with endodontic therapy. J Endod 18(10):509–511
16. Nixdorf DR, Moana-Filho EJ, Law AS et al (2010) Frequency of nonodontogenic pain after endodontic therapy: a systematic review and meta-analysis. J Endod 36(9):1494–1498
17. Polycarpou N, Ng YL, Canavan D et al (2005) Prevalence of persistent pain after endodontic treatment and factors affecting its occurrence in cases with complete radiographic healing. Int Endod J 38(3):169–178
18. Replogle K, Reader A, Nist R et al (1997) Anesthetic efficacy of the intraosseous injection of 2 % lidocaine (1:100,000 epinephrine) and 3 % mepivacaine in mandibular first molars. Oral Surg Oral Med Oral Pathol Oral Radiol Endod 83(1):30–37
19. Rosenberg PA (2003) Clinical strategies for managing endodontic pain. Endod Top 3:78–92
20. Rosenberg PA, Frisbie J, Lee J et al (2010) Evaluation of pathologists (histopathology) and radiologists (cone beam computed tomography) differentiating radicular cysts from granulomas. J Endod 36(3):423–428
21. Sathorn C, Parashos P, Messer HH (2005) Effectiveness of single- versus multiple-visit endodontic treatment of teeth with apical periodontitis: a systematic review and meta-analysis. Int Endod J 38(6):347–355
22. Woda A, Salter MW (2008) Mechanisms of neuropathic pain. Quintessence, Chicago
23. Wright EF (2000) Referred craniofacial pain patterns in patients with temporomandibular disorder. J Am Dent Assoc 131(9):1307–1315
24. Zhang J, Kawashima N, Suda H et al (2006) The existence of CD11c+ sentinel and F4/80+ interstitial dendritic cells in dental pulp and their dynamics and functional properties. Int Immunol 18(9):1375–1384

2 Odontogenic and Non-odontogenic Pain

2.1 Terminology: Basic Pain Biology

2.1.1 Peripheral Nervous System

Most often pain is caused by tissue damage, or the potential for tissue damage, and is transmitted via terminal nerve fibers known as primary afferent nerve fibers to higher centers.

Two major classes of nociceptive (or pain-sensing) primary afferent nerve fibers can detect potentially damaging noxious stimuli: the A-delta and C fibers. Both fiber types have a wide distribution throughout the body including the dental pulp. In addition, separate classes of nerve fibers exist that are involved in detecting non-noxious stimuli such as vibration and proprioception. Such fibers can be found in the periodontal ligament, skin, and oral mucosa and include the A-beta fibers [13].

2.1.2 Primary Afferent Neurons

In the peripheral nervous system, neurons or nerves are referred to as primary afferent (i.e., sensory) fibers. The primary afferent fibers can be divided broadly into A-beta fibers, which transmit light touch or proprioceptive information, and A-delta and C fibers, which encode pain. The tooth is richly innervated by afferent nerve fibers, which are believed to primarily transmit pain in response to thermal, mechanical, or chemical stimuli. The vast majority of dental nerves are C fibers that innervate the central pulp, most of which terminate beneath the odontoblasts [6].

2.1.3 A-Beta Fibers

Rapidly conducting myelinated neurons that respond to light touch are called A-beta fibers. Under normal conditions, activation of the A-beta fibers by

P.A. Rosenberg, *Endodontic Pain*,
DOI 10.1007/978-3-642-54701-0_2, © Springer-Verlag Berlin Heidelberg 2014

high-intensity stimulation results in low-frequency output in the central nervous system. Activation of A-beta fibers normally is interpreted as non-painful mechanical stimulation [15] or "pre-pain" [6]. A-beta fibers have been shown to undergo phenotypic changes that allow them to encode painful stimuli under inflammatory conditions [19].

2.1.4 A-Delta Fibers

A-delta fibers are lightly myelinated, have a faster conduction velocity than C fibers, and are believed to transmit a sharp or pricking sensation. A-delta fibers respond primarily to noxious mechanical stimuli rather than to chemical or thermal stimuli. Other A-delta fibers may be polymodal (responding to mechanical, chemical, and thermal stimuli) [3] or respond only to cold/mechanical [15] or hot/mechanical noxious stimuli [10].

In the dental pulp, A-delta fibers cross the odontoblastic layer and terminate in the dentinal tubules [13]. Due to their location and their sensitivity to mechanical stimulation, A-delta fibers are believed to respond to stimuli that result in movement of fluid within the dentinal tubules (e.g., osmotic, mechanical probing, or thermal stimuli applied to the external surface of the tooth) [13]. Consistent with that theory of dentinal pain is the fact that the stimuli causing dentinal fluid movement result in sharp pain associated with A-delta fiber activation. When intense noxious stimuli activate the A-delta fibers, the input to the central nervous system consists of high-frequency action potentials.

2.1.5 C Fibers

C fibers are unmyelinated, have slower conduction velocity, and are associated with a dull, aching, or burning sensation. Most C fibers respond to mechanical, thermal, and chemical stimuli. Because of the difference in conduction velocities, A-delta fibers are believed to transmit early shooting pain, while C fibers transmit late, dull pain.

Noxious stimuli that exceed the receptor threshold of these nociceptive primary afferent terminals result in action potentials that travel centrally, signaling tissue damage. In the pulp tissue, the more centrally located C fibers respond to thermal, mechanical, and chemical stimuli and are believed to be sensitized by inflammation [10]. All visceral structures are innervated primarily by afferent fibers conducting nociceptive information such as that carried by A-delta and C fibers [13].

2.1.6 Allodynia and Hyperalgesia

Allodynia and hyperalgesia are two different pain entities characterized by an increased patient response to painful stimuli. In some situations they can occur shortly after pain stimuli or take some time to develop.

2.1.7 Allodynia

Allodynia is defined as a reduction in pain threshold so that previously non-noxious stimuli are perceived as painful.

A classic example is an experience with sunburn. Following sunburn simply wearing a shirt can cause pain. This is an example of a reduced pain threshold (allodynia), resulting in pain from a stimulus that would not normally be painful. If someone gently touches the burned skin, the result may be sudden severe pain.

During irreversible pulpitis simply touching a tooth or exerting pressure on it may be enough to provoke pain. Allodynia focuses on a reduced pain threshold. This is an example of increased pain perception (hyperalgesia) caused by a stimulus that would not normally be painful [13].

2.1.8 Hyperalgesia

Hyperalgesia may be defined as an increase in the perceived magnitude of a painful stimulus. The focus in this condition is on the disproportionate reaction to a stimulus. If a patient has pulp/periapical pathosis, they may experience severe pain from gentle tapping a tooth with pericementitis. This is an example of both a reduced pain threshold (allodynia) and an increased pain perception (hyperalgesia.)

Clinicians often rely on clinical testing and the patient's symptoms to detect the presence of hyperalgesia and allodynia. These are important symptoms associated with irreversible pulpitis [13].

Hyperalgesia can be partially accounted for by sensitization of nociceptors (primary hyperalgesia) and by central nervous system mechanisms (secondary hyperalgesia).

In the absence of tissue damage, activation of C or A-delta fibers produces transient pain. This pain is believed to serve as a physiological warning. When there is tissue injury, afferent fibers may be activated by lower-intensity stimuli than usual, and the quality of pain may be more persistent and intense. This phenomenon is due, in part, to sensitization of nociceptors, including an increase in spontaneous activity.

At the site of tissue injury, there are a number of inflammatory mediators that can directly or indirectly sensitize primary afferent nociceptors. These inflammatory mediators may be released from the local tissue cells, circulating and resident immune cells, vasculature and endothelial smooth muscle cells, and peripheral nervous system cells [13].

2.1.9 Central Sensitization

After peripheral tissue injury there is an afferent barrage from C fibers resulting from peripheral tissue inflammation, decreased afferent thresholds, and spontaneous firing of afferent fibers. When a second-order neuron receives a prolonged barrage of nociceptive input, the second-order neuron may also become sensitized. This results in a phenomenon referred to as central sensitization. The result of central sensitization is enhanced processing (i.e., amplification) of neural impulses that are being transmitted to higher brain centers. Two effects of central sensitization are secondary hyperalgesia and referred pain [13].

Secondary hyperalgesia is an increased response to painful stimulation at the site of pain resulting from central nervous system changes. This is in contrast to primary hyperalgesia, which is a lowered pain threshold resulting from sensitization of peripheral neurons. Secondary hyperalgesia might be felt in superficial (e.g., gingiva or skin) or deep structures (e.g., muscles or teeth).

2.1.10 Peripheral Sensitization

After tissue insult there is an inflammatory reaction that often causes pain. The severity of pain that follows is related to several aspects of the injury. Important are the type, extent, and location of the injury; the innervation of the tissue; and the phase of the inflammation. In the nociceptive system, tissue injury can manifest itself as increased responsiveness and/or reduced thresholds to a noxious stimulus, referred to as hyperalgesia [13].

2.2 Recognizing "What the Pain Is Not"

Often, a dentist feels under pressure to develop a precise diagnosis for the cause of pain, but that may not always be possible. It is critical that the dentist recognizes the significance of clues provided in the history and by clinical examination. While the dentist may not be able to synthesize the information and diagnose the precise cause of pain, it is possible that pulp/periapical can be *ruled out*. This is a critical point in the diagnostic process and leads the inquiry in a different direction.

Recognizing that the cause of pain is non-odontogenic is a crucial finding. The patient's complaint of tooth-based pain may be misleading. When it becomes clear that the cause is non-odontogenic, a different path of inquiry is required. In diagnostically challenging cases, the astute diagnostician recognizes when it is wise to reach out to others for assistance. For example, referral to an endodontist, an orofacial pain specialist, or neurologist can be helpful in establishing the precise cause of pain. Failure to reach an evidence-based diagnosis increases the possibility of unnecessary treatment.

When the diagnosis is unclear, and the patient is not in severe pain, the clinician may have the option of delaying the definitive diagnosis and treatment plan. Often, symptoms will localize in the days or weeks following an initial visit and that transition facilitate the diagnostic process. In contrast, if the patient is in severe pain and diagnostic tests do not provide a clear diagnosis, the dentist should describe the situation to the patient and provide reasonable options including the possibility of referral. The patient must be brought into the decision making process in order to avoid potential unpleasantness if the treatment provided turns out to be in error.

> Wise Advice
> "You can see a lot just by listening."
> Yogi Berra
> American baseball player and humorist

2.2.1 Odontogenic Toothache

Pulpal pain is mediated by C fibers and may be described as dull, aching, or throbbing in nature. This is in contrast to the quick short sharp sensation produced by A-delta fibers that mediate dentinal pain. When pulp testing, it is important to note not only whether the patient perceived the stimulus but also the nature of the stimulus perceived.

Pulp inflammation can result in sensitization of nerve fibers. When peripheral nociceptors (e.g., pulpal C fibers) are sensitized, the threshold of firing in response to a given stimulus (e.g., temperature and pressure) is lowered. In states of sensitization these nociceptors can be provoked with a less intense stimulus. The threshold for excitation is still "all or nothing," but the required level of stimulation has decreased. These factors are involved in development of what is termed a "hot tooth," and its management is discussed in Chap. 6 [13].

Unlike pulpal pain, pain of periradicular origin is easier to localize. Mechanoreceptors are numerous in the periodontal ligament (PDL) and are most densely concentrated in the apical third [17]. When inflammation from pulpal disease extends into the periodontal ligament, patients are more able to locate the source of the pain [13].

Clinical Tips

- Gently tapping a suspect tooth with a mirror handle (or even just finger pressure against a highly sensitive tooth) is an excellent means of confirming a patient's complaint.
- A painful response to percussion is an indication of inflammation of the periodontal ligament and is termed pericementitis.
- In the absence of a new restoration in hyper-occlusion or acute periodontal disease, pericementitis is an indication of pulpitis extending into the periapical tissue.
- In the presence of sensitivity to percussion, treatment often involves endodontic therapy including occlusal reduction.

The degree of discomfort that a patient feels in relation to their periradicular pain is dependent on the degree of peripheral sensitization and the amount of provocation to this structure. A sensitized PDL will be uncomfortable to a patient if percussed lightly but more uncomfortable if percussed heavily. This is known as a graded response [13].

It is helpful to record the results of periradicular testing such as percussion and palpation in terms of degrees of tenderness (vs. "all or nothing"). Even using simple numerical values such as +1, +2, +3 provides useful information if a patient must return for a second diagnostic visit. See pain scale Fig. 1.1. As with pulpal pain, pain of periradicular origin should also have an identifiable etiology.

Heterotopic Pain (Referred Pain)

Most patients reporting dental pain have symptoms that are odontogenic. However, the site the patient feels pain may not be the actual source of pain. Although patients may perceive that pain originates in a specific tooth, the pain may actually be referred from non-dental structures. Similarly, dental pain may be referred to non-dental structures.

The dentist must start the diagnostic process recognizing that a significant percentage of patient's reports concerning the origin of pain are erroneous. Initiating endodontic treatment without confirmatory tests can lead to unnecessary treatment and continued pain. See Chaps. 1 and 6 for further discussion.

2.2.2 Non-odontogenic Pain

Pain of Sinus and/or Nasal Mucosal Origin

Pain of sinus and/or nasal mucosal origin is discussed in Chap. 1, but it is mentioned again here because it is a classic example of heterotopic pain (referred pain).

Myofascial Pain

Patients often describe myofascial pain as deep, dull, and aching, and it can be associated with referred dental pain. It has been demonstrated that three masticatory muscles commonly refer pain to teeth. The muscles are the superior belly of the masseter (to the maxillary posterior teeth) and inferior belly of the masseter (to mandibular posterior teeth), the temporal (to maxillary anterior or posterior teeth), and the mandibular to the mandibular anterior teeth (Figs. 2.1, 2.2, 2.3, 2.4, 2.5, 2.6, 2.7, 2.8, and 2.9) [22].

Headache Disorders

Of most interest to dental clinicians are the primary headache disorders, which comprise the bulk of those disorders, and may present as non-odontogenic toothaches. They can be grouped as migraine, tension headache, and cluster headache.

Migraine

Patients may report a history of migraine headaches. This is useful information and leads the clinician to a process of differential diagnosis directed at

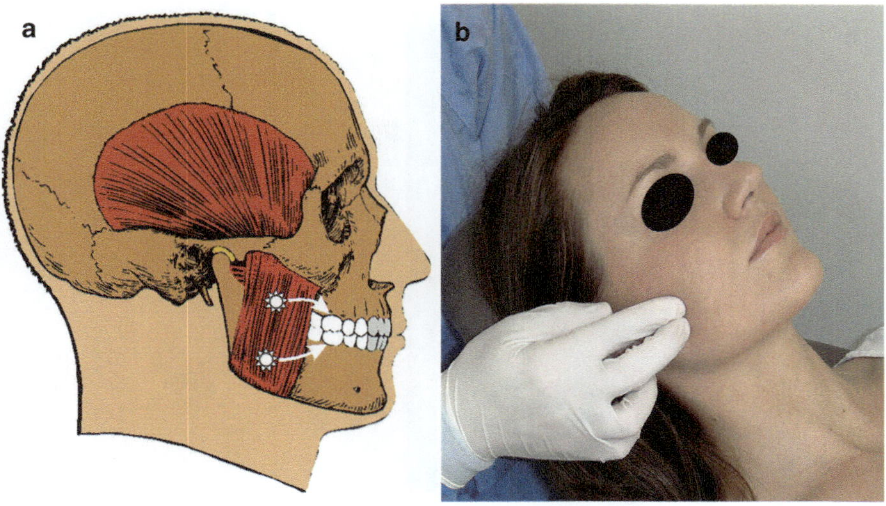

Fig. 2.1 (a) Trigger points in the masseter muscle can refer any pain to the maxillary or mandibular posterior teeth. (b) Palpation of the masseter muscle to assess for any pain that may be referred to the posterior tooth (Reproduced from Seltzer and Bender's Dental Pulp)

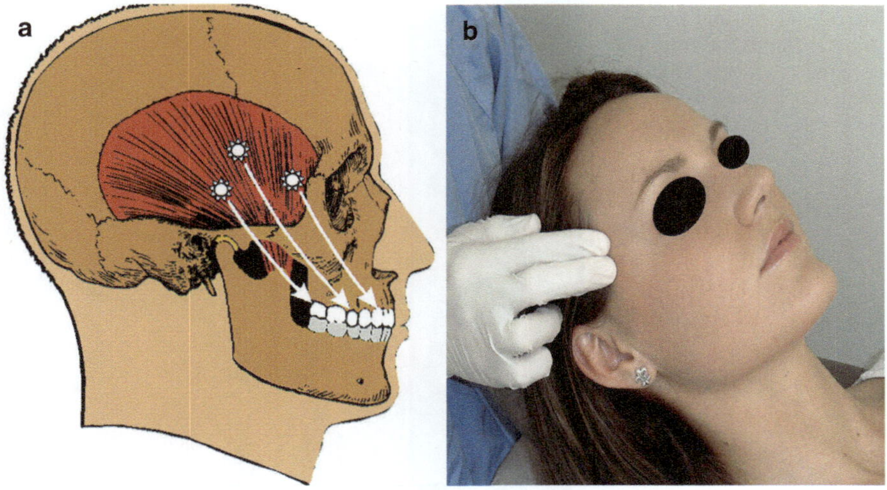

Fig. 2.2 (a) Trigger points in the temporalis muscle can refer pain to the maxillary teeth. (b) Palpation of the temporalis muscle to assess for any pain that may be referred to the maxillary teeth (Reproduced from Seltzer and Bender's Dental Pulp)

differentiating pulp/periapical pain from headache pain. Symptoms such as an aura, nausea, vomiting, and photophobia or phonophobia are indicators of non-endodontic pain.

Migraine is a common headache, with about 18 % of females and 6 % of males experiencing this type of headache [16, 23]. It is associated with significant amounts

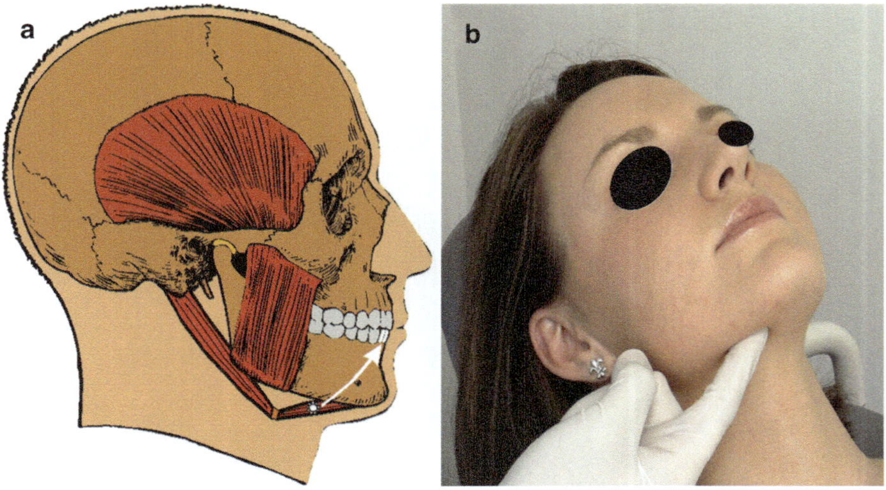

Fig. 2.3 (**a**) Trigger points in the anterior digastric muscle can refer pain to mandibular anterior teeth. (**b**) Palpation of the anterior belly of the digastric muscle to assess for any pain that may be referred to the mandibular anterior teeth (Reproduced from Seltzer and Bender's Dental Pulp)

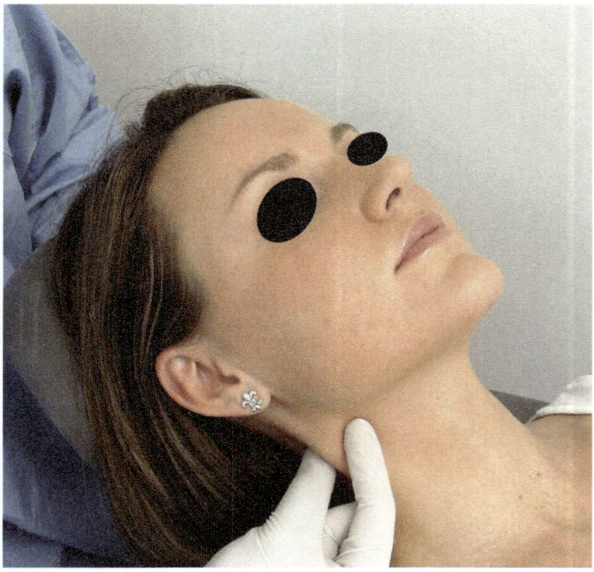

Fig. 2.4 Palpation of the sternocleidomastoid muscle to assess for pain that may be referred to the face, TMJ, or teeth (Reproduced from Seltzer and Bender's Dental Pulp)

of disability, which is the motivating factor that brings the patient to seek care and the reason why this type of headache is the one most often seen in medical clinics.

Migraine has been reported to present as toothache [1, 8] and is likely the most common neurovascular disorder to do so. In addition to this, people with migraine headaches are thought of as having increased regional pain sensitivity that has diagnostic and treatment implications for the clinician [20].

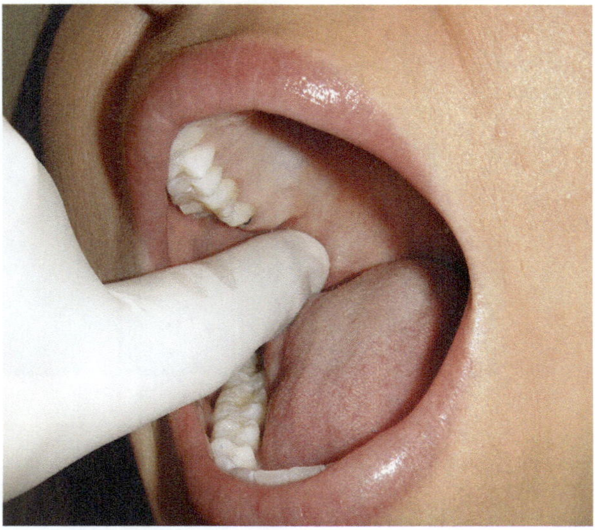

Fig. 2.5 Intra oral palpation of the medial pterygoid muscle in order to assess for pain that may be referred to posterior teeth (Reproduced from Hargreaves et al. [13])

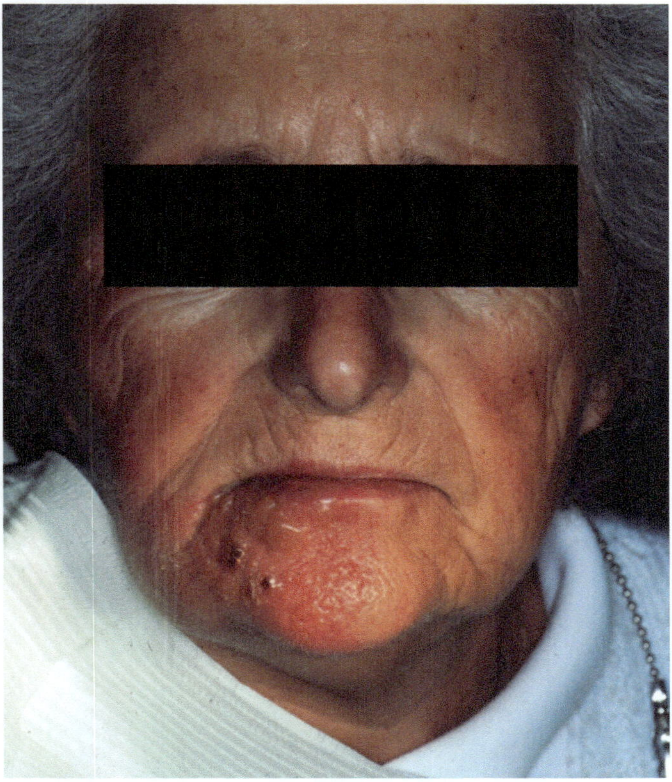

Fig. 2.6 Patient complained of vague discomfort, mandibular right side

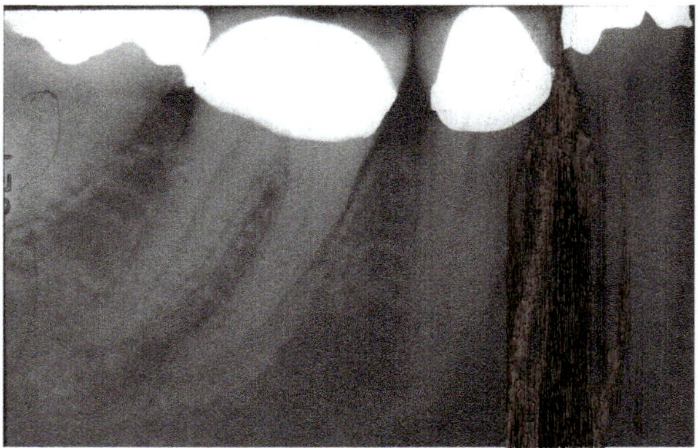

Fig. 2.7 Radiograph. Patient focused on mandibular right first premolar as the cause of her pain

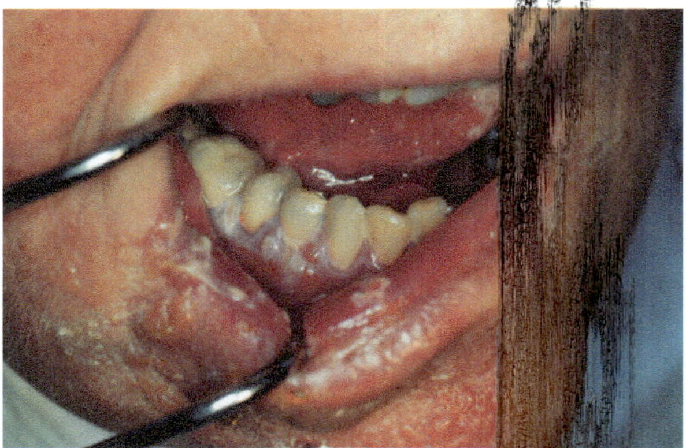

Fig. 2.8 Four days later initial appearance of intraoral lesions

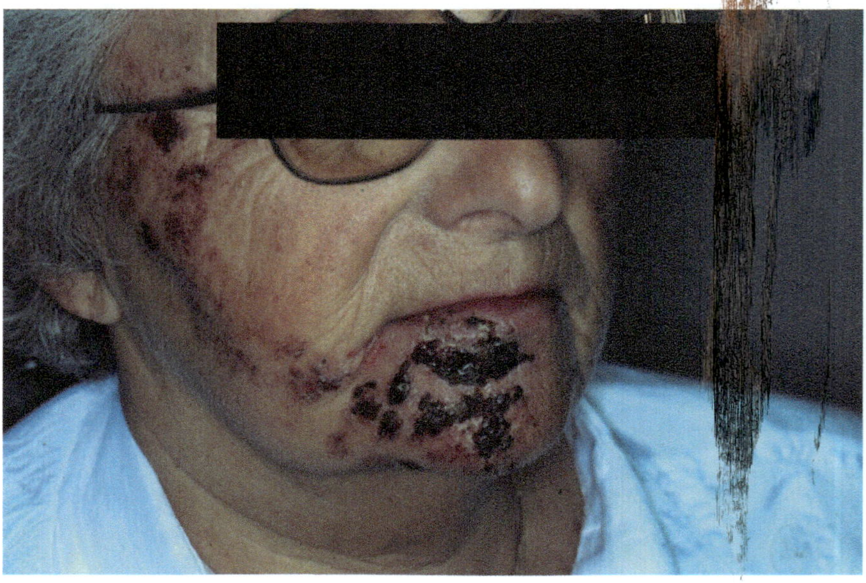

Fig. 2.9 Twenty-five days after initiation of symptoms (Courtesy of Dr. Asgeir Sigurdsson)

Migraine headaches typically last between 4 and 72 h. They tend to be unilateral in presentation and pulsatile in quality, with a moderate to severe intensity of pain. Patients may also experience nausea and/or vomiting, as well as photophobia or phonophobia, which are different from toothache. The headache is usually aggravated with routine physical activity, such as walking up stairs.

Caffeine/ergotamine compounds have been used widely in the past as abortive agents for migraine headaches, but in contemporary times they have been replaced with triptans, such as sumatriptan and rizatriptan [18]. Migraine headaches may partially or fully abate with the use of nonsteroidal anti-inflammatory medications in a similar fashion as toothaches [13].

Tension Headache

Tension-type headache is the most frequent headache disorder experienced, with a range of reported prevalence from 41 to 96 %. The wide range can be attributed to varied definitions of tension headache.

Tension-type headaches may be a heterogeneous group of similarly presenting head pains that have overlapping pathophysiologic mechanisms, which has led some researchers to consider aspects of tension-type headache to be the same as musculoskeletal orofacial pain, known as temporomandibular disorders (TMDs) [13].

Cluster Headache

Cluster headaches and other TACs (trigeminal autonomic cephalgias) are rare neurovascular painful disorders that are unilateral and defined by the concurrent presentation of at least one ipsilateral autonomic symptom such as nasal congestion, rhinorrhea, lacrimation, eyelid edema, periorbital swelling, facial erythema, ptosis, or miosis that occurs with the pain [13].

The major distinguishing features between these headache disorders are the duration and frequency of the pain episodes, as well as the gender most often afflicted. Cluster headache is the most common of the group, occurring in men three to four times more often than in women, with pain episodes lasting between 15 min and 2 h that occur at a frequency of eight episodes per day to one every other day. These headaches occur in clusters, with active periods of 2 weeks to 3 months.

Clinical Tips

- Elimination of pain after 10 min inhalation of 100 % oxygen is diagnostic for cluster headache [13].

From a non-odontogenic perspective, cluster headache and almost all the other TACs have been reported to present as non-odontogenic toothache.

The concurrent autonomic features, such as discoloration or swelling in the anterior maxilla, might compound the diagnostic problem by suggesting tooth abscess. Neurovascular headaches tend to be episodic with complete remission between episodes, while odontogenic pain usually has at least some background pain that stays between exacerbations. Local anesthetic is unpredictable in these cases and can mislead the clinician.

Initial management by dentists is aimed at determining whether or not the pain is of odontogenic origin. If it is not of odontogenic origin, the patient should then be referred to an appropriate care provider [13].

2.2.3 Neuralgia

The term "neuralgia" when used generically to describe intraoral pain can lead to confusion. The word neuralgia may be used to refer to what is thought of as classic trigeminal neuralgia or tic douloureux. The term "neuralgia" may be used to describe pain felt along a specific peripheral nerve distribution, such as with postherpetic neuralgia and occipital neuralgia, as opposed to a focus of pain disorders that have similar characteristics and are thought to have common underlying pathophysiologic mechanisms [13].

Trigeminal neuralgia is characteristically an intense, sharp shooting pain that is most often unilateral. There is usually an area that, on stimulation such as light touch, elicits sharp shooting pain. The area that elicits the pain is referred to as a trigger zone, and it can be in the distribution of the resultant pain or in a different distribution—but is always ipsilateral. Most patients present with a characteristic trigger zone, but not all patients will present with this finding [13].

An important characteristic of trigger zones is that the response to the stimulus is not proportional to the intensity of the stimulus. That is, slight pressure on a trigger zone results in severe pain. In addition, once triggered, pain typically subsides within a few minutes until triggered again. This is in contrast to odontogenic pain, which may come and go but does not do so in such a predictable and repeatable manner. The trigger for odontogenic pain is an area that has no sensory abnormalities (e.g., dysesthesia or paresthesia) [13].

Because symptoms can be quite severe, patients may insist on treatment even though the clinical findings do not support an odontogenic etiology. The misleading symptoms, along with the willingness of the patient to consent to

Clinical Tips

- Sharp shooting pain in the absence of a dental etiology associated with the symptoms (e.g., caries, large restorations, dental trauma, or recent dental treatment) should alert the clinician to consider trigeminal neuralgia in the differential diagnosis.
- These patients should be referred to a neurologist or orofacial pain specialist in order to confirm the diagnosis.

endodontic treatment, emphasize the importance of a thorough history and clinical evaluation.

Herpes Zoster (Shingles)

Ninety percent of the US population has serologic evidence of varicella infection and is at risk for the development of herpes zoster [21]. Approximately one in three people will develop zoster during their lifetime resulting in approximately one million episodes in the United States annually [13].

Neuritis is a condition caused by inflammation of a nerve or nerves secondary to injury or infection of viral or bacterial etiology. In general, pain from a virally induced neuritis, such as recurrent herpes simplex or herpes zoster, is associated with skin or mucosal lesions. Neuritic pain typically is a persistent, non-pulsatile burning and is often associated with sensory aberrations such as paresthesia, dysesthesia, or anesthesia. The pain can vary in intensity, but when stimulated, the pain provoked is disproportionate to the stimulus [13].

Because neuritic disorders are caused by reactivation of a virus that has been dormant in the trigeminal ganglion, they are considered projected pain with distribution within the dermatomes innervated by the affected peripheral nerves. In some cases, there may not be cutaneous lesions because the nerves affected by the virus may supply deeper tissues [13].

Clinical Tips

- Herpes zoster may present a diagnostic challenge if pain precedes the outbreak of vesicles on the mucus membrane or skin [9].
- Patients in this group may present with severe oral pain that cannot be localized to a specific tooth. This can lead to unnecessary endodontic treatment of a suspect tooth.

Localized traumatic injury can also induce neuritis. This injury can be chemical, thermal, or mechanical in nature. A classic endodontic example of a chemical injury to a nerve is the overextension of a highly neurotoxic paraformaldehyde-containing paste (e.g., Sargenti paste) onto the inferior alveolar nerve. Chemical trauma can be due to certain toxic components of the endodontic filling materials such as eugenol, irrigating solutions such as sodium hypochlorite, or intra-canal medicaments such as formocresol.

Mechanical compression in addition to thermal trauma may be a factor when thermoplasticized material, or carrier-based material, results in overextension of the filling. Mechanical nerve trauma is more commonly associated with oral surgery procedures such as orthognathic surgery and third molar extraction.

Clinical Tips

- The zoster vaccine reduces the incidence of herpes zoster by approximately 50 % and the occurrence of postherpetic neuralgia by two thirds, with vaccinated individuals experiencing attenuated or shortened symptoms.
- The zoster vaccine should be offered to most individuals older than 60 years of age [21].

Recent Research

A retrospective study in the United Kingdom reported that having shingles may increase the risk of having a stroke years later, according to research published online in the January 2, 2014 online issue of Neurology, The American Academy of Neurology.

People aged 14–40 who had shingles were more likely to have a stroke, heart attack, or transient ischemic attack (TIA) than those who had not had shingles.

The study determined that people under 40 years of age were 74 % more likely to have a stroke if they had had shingles, after adjusting for stroke risk factors such as obesity, smoking, and high cholesterol.

People under 40 years of age were 50 % more likely to have a heart attack if they had shingles.

The numbers differed in those over 40 years of age. For example, in that group people were 15 % more likely to have a heart attack if they had shingles [5].

Neuropathy

The term neuropathy describes localized, sustained non-episodic pain secondary to an injury or change in a neural structure. Atypical facial pain is included in this category. This term suggests pain that is felt in a branch of the trigeminal nerve and that does not fit any other pain category [8, 12].

If a misdiagnosis occurs a tooth may unnecessarily be extracted. Unfortunately, if the pain is due to non-odontogenic causation, the pain will persist and is then referred to as phantom tooth pain. A limitation in the use of the terms "atypical facial pain" and "phantom tooth pain" is that they suggest that there is pain of unknown etiology, and there is a lack of information regarding their pathophysiology [13].

Psychogenic Toothache

A patient may complain of dental pain (a somatic complaint) without an actual cause. This situation is included in a category of psychogenic toothache that is a psychological disorder. Psychogenic toothache falls within a group of mental disorders known as somatoform. The word "somatoform" is derived from the fact that while the patient has somatic complaints, there is a lack of physical cause. Because these patients lack a physical cause for pain, they will present without local tissue changes. Patients with somatoform disorder are not fabricating the symptoms, nor are they seeking conscious benefit. It is important to make a distinction between somatoform disorders and factitious or malingering disorders [13].

Psychogenic pain may be caused by severe psychological stress. These pains present a general departure from the characteristics of any other pain condition. That is, they may not fit normal anatomic distributions or physiological patterns. The pain may be felt in multiple teeth, and the pain may jump around from one tooth to another. The intensity of pain tends to be more severe than is reflected by the patient's level of concern about their condition. Their response to therapy is variable, including a lack of response or an unusual or expected response. Early identification of psychogenic pain and referral to a psychologist or psychiatrist is necessary to avoid irreversible and unnecessary dental treatment [13].

Cardiac and Thoracic Structures

Cardiac pain has been cited as the cause of non-odontogenic toothache in a number of case reports [2, 11, 14]. Classically, cardiac pain presents as a crushing substernal pain that most commonly radiates to the left arm, shoulder, neck, and face.

Although not as common, anginal pain may present solely as dental pain, generally felt in the lower left jaw. Similar to pain of pulpal origin, cardiac pain can be spontaneous and diffuse with a cyclic pattern that fluctuates in intensity from mild to severe. The pain can also be intermittent, and the patient may be completely asymptomatic at times. The quality of cardiac pain when referred to the mandible is chiefly aching and sometimes pulsatile.

Cardiac pain may be spontaneous or increased with physical exertion, emotional upset, or even the ingestion of food [2]. Cardiac pain cannot be aggravated by local provocation of teeth. Anesthetizing the lower jaw or providing dental treatment will not reduce the pain. It can be decreased with rest or a dose of sublingual nitroglycerin. Diagnosis of cardiac pain, along with immediate referral, is mandatory to avoid impending myocardial infarction [13].

Besides pain of cardiac origin, other chest structures have been reported to produce non-odontogenic toothache pain. Various cancerous lesions of the lungs have been described to present a mandibular pain, on both the ipsilateral and contralateral sides of the tumor [7], as well as diaphragmatic pain mediated via the phrenic nerve [4, 13].

Clinical Tips

- Complex diagnoses may require input from other health-care professionals.
- It is never a mistake to seek collaboration during the diagnostic process.

References

1. Alonso AA, Nixdorf DR (2006) Case series of four different headache types presenting as tooth pain. J Endod 32(11):1110–1113
2. Batchelder BJ, Krutchkoff DJ, Amara J (1987) Mandibular pain as the initial and sole clinical manifestation of coronary insufficiency: report of case. J Am Dent Assoc 115(5): 710–712
3. Besson JM, Chaouch A (1987) Peripheral and spinal mechanisms of nociception. Physiol Rev 67(1):67–186
4. Blows WT (1999) Diaphragmatic cramp as a possible cause of noncardiac chest pain and referred mandibular pain. J Neurosci Nurs 31(3):187–190
5. Breuer J, Pacou M (2014) Herpes zoster as a risk factor for stroke and TIA. Neurology 82(3):206–212
6. Brown AC, Beeler WJ, Kloka AC et al (1985) Spatial summation of pre-pain and pain in human teeth. Pain 21(1):1–16
7. Buddery DJ (2003) Mandible pain. Br Dent J 194(3):121
8. Dodick DW (2007) Migraine with isolated facial pain: a diagnostic challenge. Cephalalgia 27(11):1199–1200
9. Dubinsky RM, Kabbani H, El-Chami Z et al (2004) Practice parameter: treatment of postherpetic neuralgia: an evidence-based report of the Quality Standards Subcommittee of the American Academy of Neurology. Neurology 63(6):959–965
10. Dubner R, Hayes RL, Hoffman DS (1980) Neural and behavioral correlates of pain in the trigeminal system. Res Publ Assoc Res Nerv Ment Dis 58:63–72
11. Durso BC, Israel MS, Janini ME et al (2003) Orofacial pain of cardiac origin: a case report. Cranio 21(2):152–153
12. Glaros AG, Urban D, Locke J (2007) Headache and temporomandibular disorders: evidence for diagnostic and behavioural overlap. Cephalalgia 27(6):542–549
13. Hargreaves KM, Cohen S, Berman LH (2011) Cohen's pathways of the pulp. Mosby Elsevier, St. Louis
14. Kreiner M, Okeson JP, Michelis V et al (2007) Craniofacial pain as the sole symptom of cardiac ischemia: a prospective multicenter study. J Am Dent Assoc 138(1):74–79
15. Lamotte RH, Lundberg LE, Torebjork HE (1992) Pain, hyperalgesia and activity in nociceptive C units in humans after intradermal injection of capsaicin. J Physiol 448:749–764
16. Lipton RB, Stewart WF, Diamond S et al (2001) Prevalence and burden of migraine in the United States: data from the American Migraine Study II. Headache 41(7):646–657

17. Long A, Loescher AR, Robinson PP (1995) A quantitative study on the myelinated fiber innervation of the periodontal ligament of cat canine teeth. J Dent Res 74(6):1310–1317
18. Mondell BE (2003) A review of the effects of almotriptan and other triptans on clinical trial outcomes that are meaningful to patients with migraine. Clin Ther 25(2):331–341
19. Neumann S, Doubell TP, Leslie T et al (1996) Inflammatory pain hypersensitivity mediated by phenotypic switch in myelinated primary sensory neurons. Nature 384(6607): 360–364
20. Nixdorf DR, Velly AM, Alonso AA (2008) Neurovascular pains: implications of migraine for the oral and maxillofacial surgeon. Oral Maxillofac Surg Clin North Am 20(2):221–235, vi–vii
21. O'connor KM, Paauw DS (2013) Herpes zoster. Med Clin North Am 97(4):503–522
22. Simons DG, Travell JG, Simons LS (1999) Travell & Simons' myofascial pain and dysfunction: the trigger point manual. Williams & Wilkins, Baltimore
23. Stewart WF, Lipton RB, Celentano DD et al (1992) Prevalence of migraine headache in the United States. Relation to age, income, race, and other sociodemographic factors. JAMA 267(1):64–69

Radiographs and Diagnostic Tests 3

3.1 Radiographs

Radiographs are an essential part of the diagnostic process. The dentist must choose between several types of radiographs including conventional, digital, and cone beam techniques. There should be a specific goal for each image while simultaneously attempting to limit the patient's exposure to radiation.

3.1.1 Periapical Radiographs

A periapical radiograph represents a basic starting point and provides an overall view of the teeth and the supporting structures in the suspect quadrant. The final diagnosis and treatment plan must not be made on the basis of a single radiograph. A slight change of angulation may allow a clinician to visualize complicating factors such as additional roots, periapical pathosis, fracture, or periodontal defect that were not apparent on the initial radiograph. A periapical radiograph should allow visualization of the entire tooth as well as adjacent teeth in the quadrant. The full extent of periapical pathosis must be visible. The relationship between root apices and the mandibular canal or maxillary sinus should be observed (Figs. 3.1, 3.2, and 3.3).

Clinical Tips

- A sharper image of a tooth results from slightly increasing vertical angulation thus foreshortening periapical radiographic images.

P.A. Rosenberg, *Endodontic Pain*,
DOI 10.1007/978-3-642-54701-0_3, © Springer-Verlag Berlin Heidelberg 2014

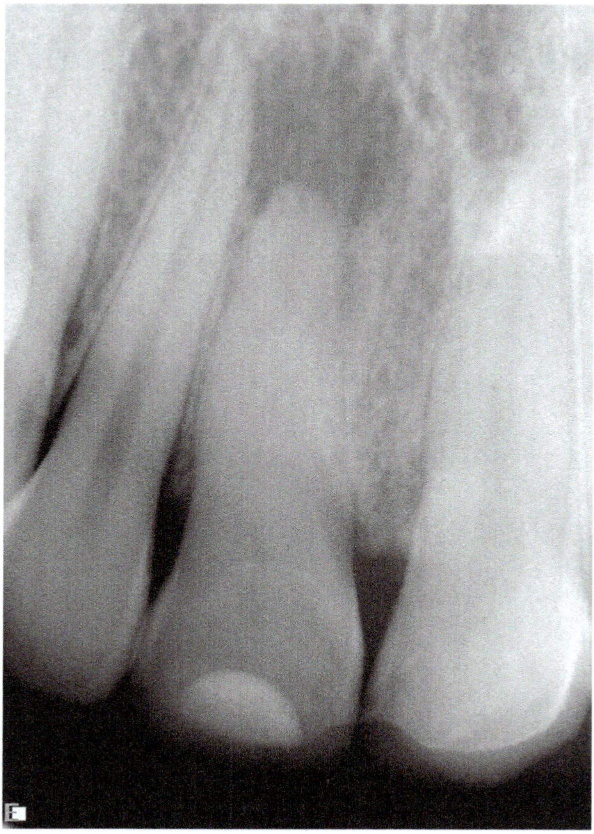

Fig. 3.1 Preoperative radiograph indicates dystrophic calcification of the canal and periapical pathosis (Courtesy of Dr. Joshua Most)

3.1.2 Bitewing Radiographs

The bitewing radiograph provides an excellent view of the pulp chamber and may reveal previous pulp caps or calcifications that were not apparent on periapical radiographs. Visualization of the pulp chamber is of value in difficult diagnostic situations. For example, a markedly constricted pulp chamber, under a deep restoration, may be evidence of long-term inflammation and calcification. This could be a valuable clue in determining the cause of a patient's pain. Visualization of the chamber is also helpful prior to establishing access. A calcified chamber makes it more challenging to establish access and identify the canals. Knowledge of a calcified chamber is important in preventing perforation of the floor of the chamber during access.

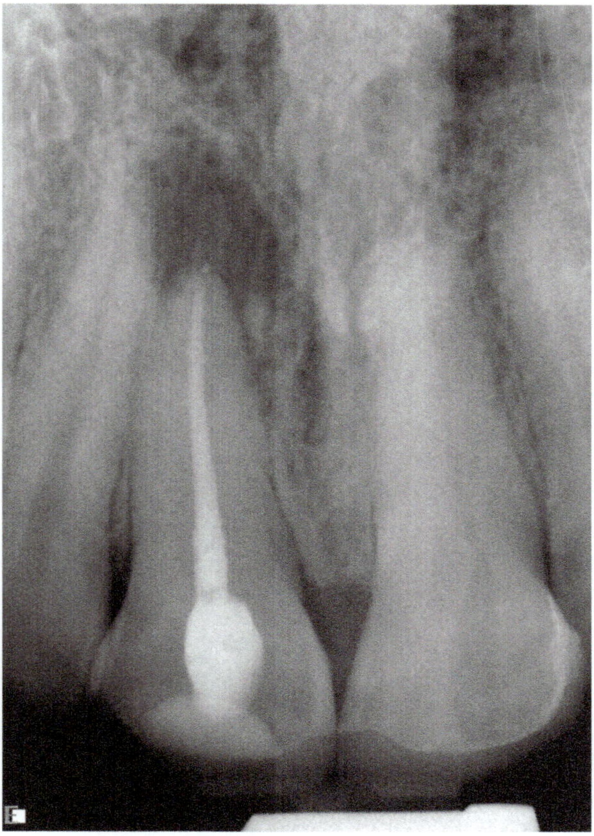

Fig. 3.2 Use of surgical operating microscope and enhanced lighting enabled treatment of the tooth (Courtesy of Dr. Joshua Most)

Clinical Tips

- Accessing a tooth with full coverage is particularly challenging because radiographs will not demonstrate chamber anatomy.
- Teeth with diffuse calcification in their chambers and full coverage are prone to perforation unless the clinician recognizes the potential problem.
- Radiographs taken before full coverage of the tooth are helpful in serving as a guide during access. The clinician is advised to develop access using slow speed after the roof of the chamber is removed. This step is helpful in preventing perforation of the chamber floor especially in teeth with full coverage or extensive restorations.

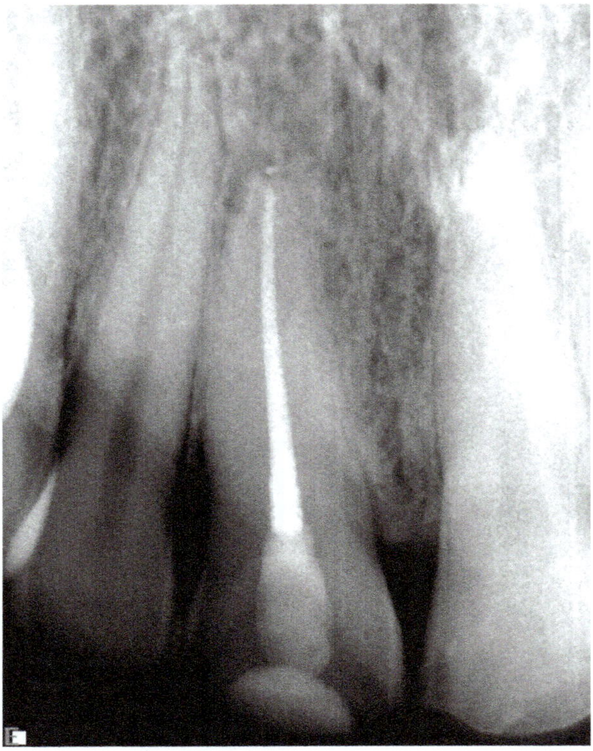

Fig. 3.3 Healed lesion (Courtesy of Dr. Joshua Most)

3.1.3 Panoramic Radiographs

Although a panoramic radiograph is useful in scanning for gross pathosis, it does not provide sufficient detail to be of value in searching for dental defects such as caries or cracks. When the clinician suspects pathosis of non-endodontic origin, it is useful in scanning the maxillae and mandible. The panoramic radiograph has been largely replaced by cone beam radiographs because of its three-dimensional capability.

3.2 Cone Beam Computed Tomography (CBCT)

The cone beam radiograph (CBCT), the newest of the radiographic modalities, has important attributes useful for an endodontist. However, it should not be used as a routine scanning device. The advantages of CBCT include three-dimensional imaging of periapical pathosis as well as canal anatomy and proximity of root apices to vital anatomic structures (Fig. 3.4).

Clinical Tips

- Three-dimensional images of periapical pathosis close to the maxillary sinus, floor of the nose, or mandibular canal are invaluable.
- A radiologist may be required to completely review a CBCT image.

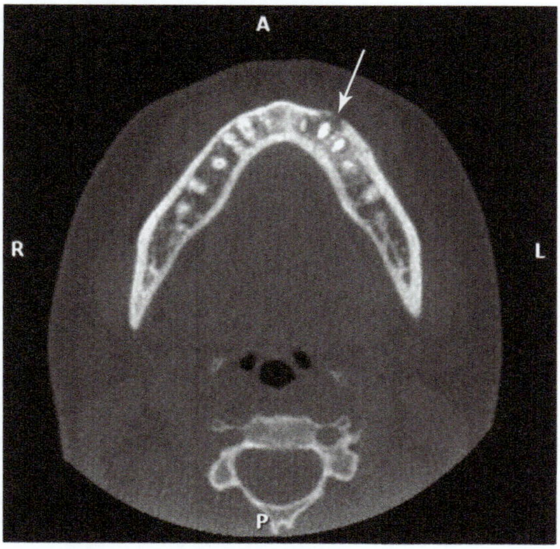

Fig. 3.4 Cone beam computed tomography (CBCT) of mandibular left premolar area. *Arrow* indicates buccal bone destruction

3.2.1 ALARA

Undue radiation exposure is a factor that must be considered. ALARA is an acronym for "as low as (is) reasonably achievable," which means making every reasonable effort to maintain patient exposure to ionizing radiation as far below the dose limits as practical [11].

3.2.2 Field of View (FOV)

Field size limitation ensures that an optimal FOV can be selected for each patient based on diagnostic needs and the region to be imaged. In general, the smaller the scan volume, the higher the resolution of the image and the lower the effective radiation dose to the patient.

3.2.3 Limited Field of View (FOV)

For most endodontic applications, limited or focused FOV CBCT is preferred over large volume CBCT for the following reasons:

- Decreased radiation exposure
- Increased resolution to improve diagnostic accuracy
- Focus on anatomic area of interest

3.2.4 Position Statement: Cone Beam Computed Tomography

The American Association of Endodontists and the American Academy of Oral and Maxillofacial Radiology jointly developed a position statement concerning cone beam computed tomography (CBCT). It is intended to provide scientifically based guidance to clinicians regarding the use of CBCT in endodontic treatment. The document, available at (www.aae.org/colleagues/), will be periodically revised to reflect new evidence [1].

3.2.5 Interpretation

Clinicians ordering a CBCT are responsible for interpreting the entire image, just as they are for any other radiographic image. Any radiograph has the potential to demonstrate findings that are significant to the health of the patient. There is no informed consent process that allows the clinician to interpret only a specific area of an image. Therefore, the clinician can be liable for a missed diagnosis, even if it is outside his/her area of practice [2]. Any questions by the practitioner regarding image data interpretation should be referred to a specialist in oral and maxillofacial radiology.

3.2.6 Recommendations

CBCT should only be used when the question for which imaging is required cannot be answered adequately by lower dose conventional dental radiography or alternate imaging modalities. Initial studies regarding the use of CBCT for a variety of endodontic-related imaging tasks have demonstrated the effectiveness and comparability of CBCT to conventional radiography [3, 7, 9, 11].

3.2.7 Research: CBCT vs. Biopsy

A study investigated the differentiation of radicular cysts from granulomas. Cone beam computed tomography (CBCT) imaging was compared with the existing standard, biopsy, and histopathology.

Based on the inconsistency of the radiologists' reports, as evidenced by statistical analyses, it was concluded that CBCT imaging is not a reliable diagnostic method for differentiating radicular cysts from granulomas.

Surgical biopsy and histopathologic evaluation remain the standard procedure for differentiating radicular cysts from granulomas [13] as well as other pathosis.

3.3 Diagnostic Testing

There are a number of sensibility tests that are useful in identifying pulp/periapical disease. Each test offers the potential of providing clues during the diagnostic process. Attempts to predict the histology of the pulp based only on clinical signs and symptoms or on electric pulp and/or thermal tests and radiographs have not been successful [5, 8].

The initial history of the chief complaint, medical and dental histories, and diagnostic radiographs represent the starting point in the inquiry and may lead the clinician to a tentative diagnosis even before sensibility tests are administered. The tests all have a degree of subjectivity associated with them, and the dentist's ability to interpret the findings is crucial.

No single test is definitive and each test should be confirmed by use of other tests. Only then can information drawn from the history of the chief complaint, radiographs, and sensibility tests be synthesized into a meaningful complete story. The pieces of the puzzle must fit. Where there is a discordant note, the clinician must reassess the evidence.

An example of a discordant note occurs when an apparent periapical lesion is associated with a root apex on radiographs but the tooth in question repeatedly tests vital on sensibility tests. A vital response to stimuli would not be expected in a tooth with a necrotic pulp and periapical pathosis. At this stage of the diagnostic process, reassessment is in order, and a non-odontogenic origin of the lesion would have to be explored.

That puzzle represents a signal to reach out for help. For example, an oral surgeon might be of assistance in performing a biopsy on the suspect lesion. A cone beam radiograph would also be helpful in providing a three-dimensional view of the lesion.

Clinical Tips
- Do not start endodontic treatment when in doubt about the origin of pain or the apparent odontogenic basis of an apical lesion.
- Recognize that commonly used diagnostic tests are subjective and can be misinterpreted.
- Depending on the results of a single test is dangerous.

3.3.1 Diagnostic Testing

This section will describe test techniques, their biological basis, and significance and the treatment indicated.

Sensibility Tests

Thermal
- Cold
- Heat
- Electric

Clinical Tests
- Palpation
- Percussion
- Bite block
- Transillumination

Assessment of pulp vitality is an important aspect of diagnosis. Responsiveness of a tooth to the application of stimuli is the basis of traditional sensibility tests [6, 8, 12]. A positive response to a sensibility test means only that there is at least some vital neural responsive tissue in the root canal. It should not be interpreted to mean that the tissue is normal or healthy.

For example, a tooth with a vital pulp and a deep carious lesion or exposure may respond normally to electric and cold sensibility tests, but that response does not indicate a healthy pulp. The clinician must interpret the results of sensibility tests with caution. These tests may be complicated by a number of clinical factors including age of the patient, recent trauma, dystrophic calcification, and the presence of large restorations. High levels of patient anxiety may also complicate the diagnostic process.

Patients' responses are subjective in nature as are the interpretations of clinicians. It is critical that clinicians recognize that there is no single definitive test. The information drawn from the history of the chief complaint, radiographs, and sensibility tests must be synthesized to reach a final diagnosis and treatment plan.

Thermal Tests

Information collected from testing with cold or heat provides an indication only of the presence or absence of functioning nerve fibers. The tests do not provide information about the blood flow and actual biological status of the tooth. A clinician may conclude that a positive response to a test means that pulp tissue is healthy, but this is not always an accurate assumption. It is advisable to consider these tests as broad screening devices that allow us to categorize teeth as vital (responsive to stimuli) or non-vital (nonresponsive). Thermal tests are divided into the application of cold and/or heat.

False-Negative and False-Positive Sensibility Tests

All sensibility tests are subject to false-positive (i.e., a positive response from a necrotic pulp) and false-negative responses (i.e., a negative response from a vital pulp) [8, 12].

One study compared results of a cold test using ethyl chloride and the outcomes of electric pulp testing to the results of endodontic access and clinical verification of pulp vitality in 59 teeth of unknown pulpal status [12]. The probability that a negative test meant a true necrotic pulp was similar for the cold and electric tests (89 % vs. 88 %): the hot gutta-percha tests exhibited a much lower ability to detect a true negative (48 %). The probability that a positive test represented a true vital pulp was similar to the cold, electric, and hot gutta-percha test (90, 84, and 83 %, respectively). Overall, the cold and electric tests had similar accuracy values (86 % vs. 81 %), and both were more accurate than the heat tests (71 %).

Other studies have reported that the cold test is more accurate (80 %) in testing human advice of more than 1,000 teeth; 2 different electric testers each resulted in approximately 5 times higher false-positive results than did the cold test. Even when gingival controls were utilized, a commercial electric tester resulted in approximately twice the number of false-positive results as compared to a cold test [5].

Good Advice
You got to be careful if you don't know where you're going, because you might not get there.

Yogi Berra
American baseball player and humorist

Responsiveness of A-delta Fibers and C Fibers

A-delta fibers are cold sensitive, and the first fibers to respond to a cold stimulus. The initial sharp pain is evoked by A-delta fibers and subsides when those fibers stop firing off. This pain is described as sharp, bright, and well localized. Temperature change causes rapid movement of fluids in the dentinal tubules that activates intratubular nerves [5].

C fibers, located deeper in the pulp, react differently. They begin to discharge after a short latency period, and their discharge rate is low. When the intradental temperature rises sufficiently, the C fibers are activated and cause a dull, throbbing, aching sensation [5].

Severe lingering response to cold, that becomes a dull ache, is considered to be a significant finding. When linked with information from the history of the chief complaint such as spontaneous pain, it is taken to be evidence of irreversible pulpitis. The results of a cold test are meaningful especially when seen in the context of the history of the chief complaint, other clinical findings, and radiographs [5].

Clinical Tips

Patients may experience transient cold sensitivity after a restorative procedure. This does not necessarily mean that the tooth has an irreversible pulpitis. Factors to consider include the severity of the pain and whether or not it lingers.

- There are limits to watchful waiting. If cold sensitivity persists over a protracted period of time, endodontic therapy is advised.
- A complex restorative procedure should not be finalized while the pulp status of a tooth is in question.

Cold Tests

There are a number of techniques for the application of cold to a tooth. Prior to testing a suspect tooth, an additional tooth serving as a control should be selected in the contralateral quadrant. The use of a control tooth allows the patient to experience a normal reaction to the stimuli prior to the actual test. The clinician is also given an opportunity to assess the responsiveness of a patient to testing of a normal pulp prior to the actual evaluation of a suspect tooth.

Ice and ethyl chloride spray have been used for many years but are not without problems. Ice is readily available, but it is only at or slightly above 0 °C, and ethyl

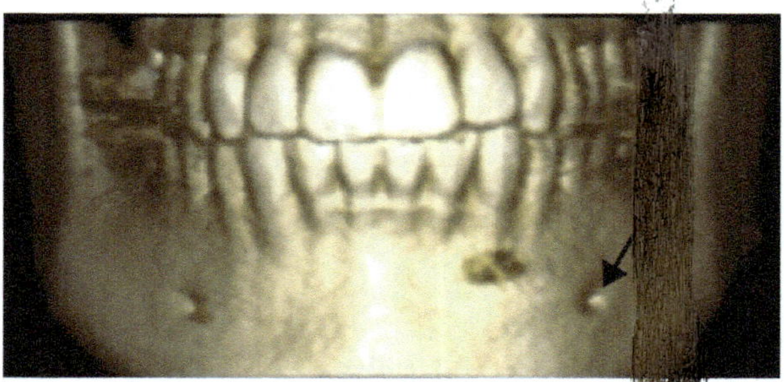

Fig. 3.5 Reconstructed image of CBCT demonstrating apical bone destruction and its relationship to the mental foramen (*arrow* points to mental foramen)

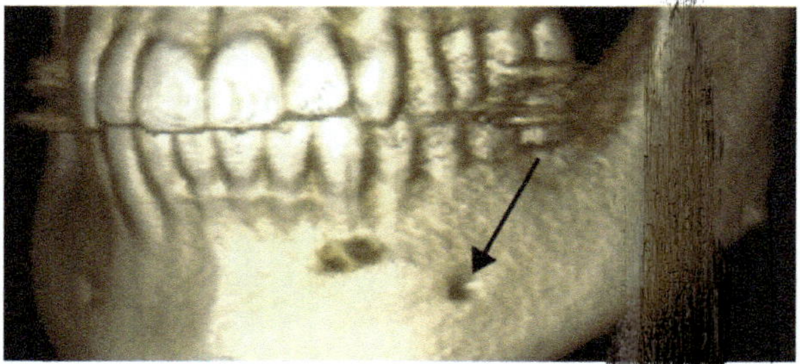

Fig. 3.6 Reconstructed image has been manipulated in order to allow a different perspective of the area. *Arrow* points to mental foramen

chloride is only about –4 °C. Cold water from melting ice can stimulate adjacent teeth and cause a misleading result. Some clinicians fill empty plastic needle cartridges with water and after freezing, and separating the two pieces have an easy-to-grip ice pencil.

Carbon dioxide pencils are also available and can be used safely on vital teeth without damaging enamel or pulp tissue [5, 10]. Carbon dioxide ice may be more reliable than ethyl chloride and ice in producing a positive response, and in young patients with incomplete root formation, carbon dioxide ice seems more reliable than electric pulp testing. [5].

Tetrafluoroethane spray has also been suggested as a test modality, but it is not as cold as carbon dioxide ice (−6.2 °C.) It is provided in cans that can be kept chair side. There appears to be no significant difference between tetrafluoroethane and carbon dioxide ice. When applying the cold stimulus, teeth should be dried and then the stimulus placed on the incisal edge or close to a pulp horn to maximize results (Figs. 3.5, 3.6 and 3.7).

Heat Tests

The application of heat can present a challenge especially in the presence of large restorations. As with cold, there is a biphasic reaction to the application of heat. A-delta fibers react first, and if a stimulus is maintained, a subsequent D fiber reaction causes a dull, radiating pain.

Several means of applying heat to a tooth have been advocated. A simple technique is to heat base plate gutta-percha until it is malleable, and then apply it to the incisal or occlusal surface of the tooth [5, 8]. Although this is a simple technique, there is no control or knowledge of the heat being applied.

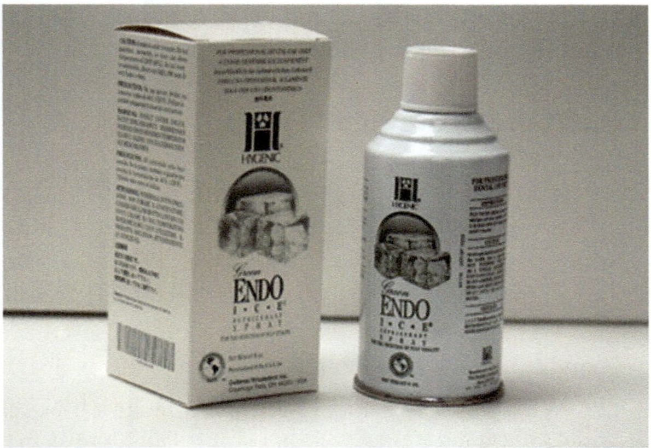

Fig. 3.7 Hygenic® Endo-Ice® Pulp Vitality Refrigerant Spray (Endo-Ice). Endo-Ice can be applied to a cotton pellet or swab for application to a tooth. It is much colder than ice or ethyl chloride at −26.2 °C. It contains no chlorofluorocarbons

Another means of applying heat is to use a dry prophylaxis cup or rubber wheel. As it rotates against the tooth, heat is generated and acts as a stimulus. Some clinicians advocate heating a plastic hand instrument and place it against the tooth in question. These rather crude techniques suffer from the same problem in terms of lack of control over the amount of teeth applied.

There is another technique that requires more time but comes closest to simulating the experience of a patient who complains of pain associated with hot fluids. With the patient in a supine position and a rubber dam in place, for isolation, a syringe is used to drip hot water on the tooth in question. The rubber dam and suction serve to prevent hot fluid from reaching adjacent teeth and protect the gingiva. Other teeth in the quadrant should be evaluated as well as the opposing arch.

No correlation has been found between an abnormal response to heat and a specific histologic diagnosis [5]. However, it is generally hypothesized that pain on heat is due to an acute irreversible pulpitis.

Some patients may present with a history of severe pain including heat sensitivity that has suddenly disappeared. Usually patients believe that the "tooth has healed" and no treatment is required. Actually, this history may be associated with devitalization of the pulp. After a period of severe pain, an asymptomatic phase may occur and is usually followed by the return of pain and swelling. Sensibility tests in such cases should indicate a lack of responsiveness.

Electric Pulp Testing

The probe should be placed as far away from the gingiva as possible, and the tooth and surrounding teeth should be dried to prevent shunting of the impulse to the gingiva. The test probe should be placed on the incisal edge or cusp tip corresponding to the pulp horn of the tooth [5].

A small amount of toothpaste or fluoride gel serves as a conducting medium [5]. The circuit must be completed with a lip contact or the patient holding the handle of the electric pulp tester. The current is started at a low value and slowly increased until the patient reports a tingling or painful sensation. As with all sensibility tests, a normal tooth, in the contralateral quadrant, should be tested first to allow the patient to understand what to expect.

Results of Electric Pulp Testing

A response to the electric stimulus indicates that there is some responsive pulp tissue present in the root canal system. It should not be interpreted to mean that the tooth is "normal" or "healthy." Research has not demonstrated a correlation between the electric pain threshold and in a pulp and histologic condition. However, no response to the test is a significant indication of pulp necrosis if the clinician can rule out factors like large restorations or dystrophic calcification of the pulp [12]. It is generally accepted that no response to an electric pulp test when associated with other findings in the history, radiographs, or clinical tests is an indication of the need for endodontic treatment.

Warning

It is not advisable to treat a tooth based solely on the results of an electric pulp test. It is well documented that results of electric pulp testing are unreliable soon after dental trauma. In teeth with incomplete root formation, the results of electric pulp testing are also not dependable [4]. There is evidence that in young teeth, cold testing is more reliable especially with carbon dioxide ice [4].

Clinical Tips

- False negatives and false-positive result can occur with all sensibility tests including electric tests.
- Always test a normal tooth in the contralateral quadrant prior to testing the tooth in question.
- Multi-rooted teeth may have responsive tissue in one canal and nonresponsive necrotic tissue in others. This could result in a false-positive response to testing.
- Confirm the test results using other sensibility and clinical tests.

Biology of Electric Pulp Testing

Electric pulp testers probably initially provoke A-delta fibers. Unmyelinated C fibers of the pulp may or may not respond [5]. There are a number of variables that may affect transmission of the impulse to the nerve fibers. Large restorations or dystrophic calcification can prevent adequate transmission of the impulse and result in a false negative response. In contrast, in a multi-rooted tooth, there may be responsive tissue in one root and nonresponsive tissue in another. A positive response will lead to a false conclusion about the status of the tooth.

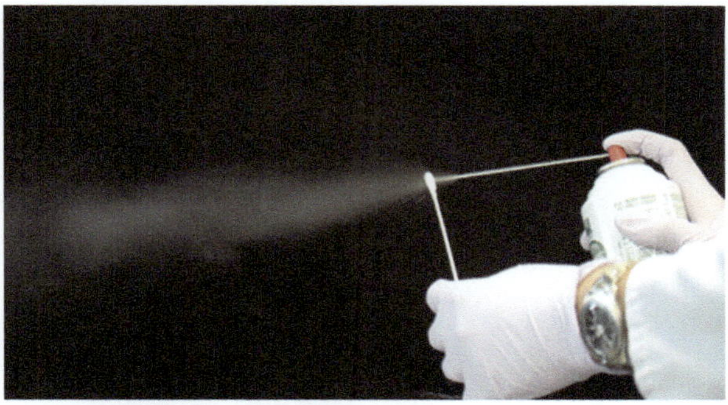

Fig. 3.8 Endo-Ice sprayed on cotton swab. Endo-Ice can be applied to a cotton pellet or swab for application to a tooth

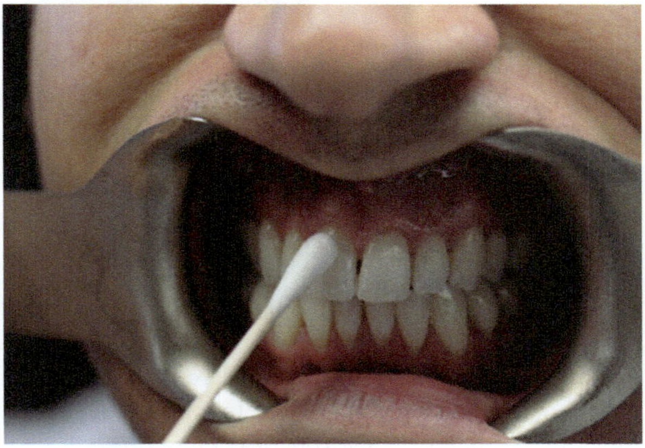

Fig. 3.9 Swab applied to tooth. Endo-Ice can be applied to a cotton pellet or swab for application to a tooth

Although there is evidence that the bipolar mode of pulp tester is more accurate because the current is confined to the coronal pulp, most electric pulp testers are monopolar [5].

3.3.2 Clinical Tests

Palpation and percussion are clinical tests that provide valuable information in addition to the results of sensibility tests. The information resulting from palpation and percussion tests should be integrated with other diagnostic data to provide a more complete view of the problem.

Palpation

This test can provide important information about the presence of inflammation in the bone and/or soft tissue overlying a root even before it appears on a radiograph. First, using a normal tooth in the contralateral quadrant, the clinician should press an index finger against the gingiva close to the margin of the crown and slowly move the finger upward (in a maxillary tooth) toward the root apex [5] (Figs. 3.8, 3.9 and 3.10).

Starting with a normal tooth provides a preview of the procedure for the patient and an opportunity for the dentist to observe the patient's reaction. Next the dentist

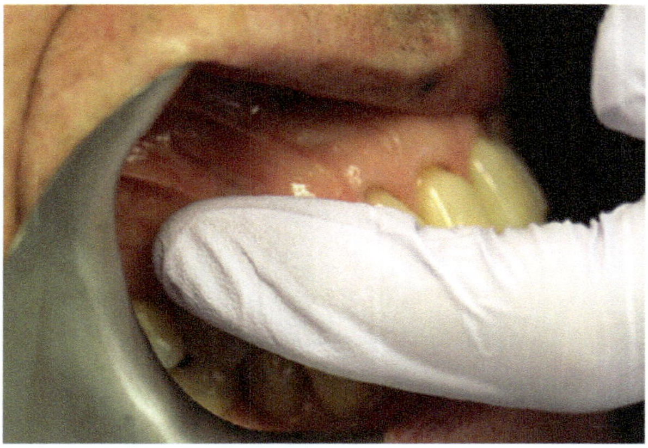

Fig. 3.10 Palpation in the gingival third of the mucobuccal fold

should move to the questionable tooth or teeth and follow the same procedure. It can also be done on the palatal or lingual surface of teeth.

Pain elicited in the gingival third is often associated with a periodontal problem, while pain in the middle third may be due to a root fracture or perforation from a post. Classically, pain in the periapical third is more likely to be associated with periapical pathosis.

However, there are numbers of variables that can affect the results of palpation. For example, in areas where the labial bone is thin, as above a maxillary canine, central incisor, or the mesiobuccal root of a maxillary first molar, palpation can provide meaningful information. In areas where the overlying bone is thicker as in mandibular molars or incisors, it is more difficult to elicit a response. If there is no response to palpation, it does not necessarily mean that periapical inflammation is absent.

The results of palpation must be interpreted carefully. For example, roots of mandibular incisors are close to each other, and sensitivity to palpation can be easily attributed to the wrong tooth. A similar situation exists in the maxillary molar area where the distobuccal root of a first molar is often quite close to the mesiobuccal root of a second molar. The results of palpation in those areas must be judged with caution.

Percussion

The percussion test can provide extremely meaningful information. The technique is quite simple. A mirror handle is usually used to gently tap the occlusal or incisal edge of a suspect tooth after first demonstrating the procedure on a normal tooth in the contralateral quadrant. For patients presenting with severe pain, gentle finger pressure should be used instead of the mirror handle [5].

Percussion of a normal tooth elicits no significant pain. Sensitivity to percussion often indicates the progression of an inflammatory process from the root canal into the periodontal ligament and adjacent tissues. It is further evidence of an irreversible pulpitis.

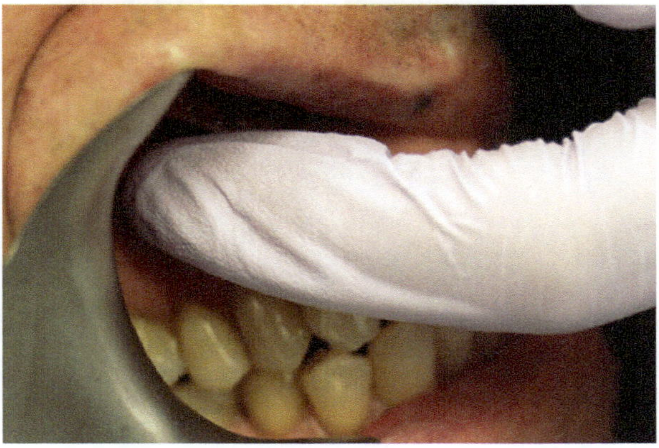

Fig. 3.11 Palpation in the middle third of the mucobuccal fold

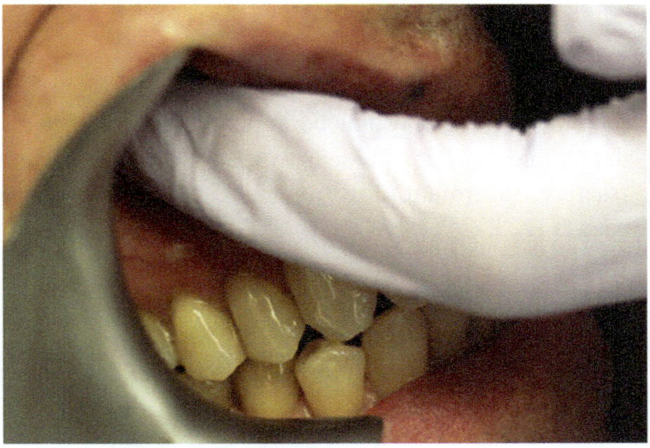

Fig. 3.12 Palpation in the apical third of the mucobuccal fold

If supraocclusion, due to a new restoration or an acute periodontal problem, can be ruled out, a positive response to percussion usually indicates extension of pulpal inflammation into the periodontal ligament and surrounding bone. Pericementitis is a common symptom indicating a need for root canal therapy.

An advantage of the percussion test is its specificity. Unlike palpation, which may not identify an individual tooth, percussion can clearly identify a painful tooth. Patients will usually be able to recognize the difference between percussing a normal tooth and the tooth in question. When a doubt exists, despite using other sensibility tests, treatment should be deferred (Figs. 3.11 and 3.12).

Clinical Tips

- Always percuss a quadrant of teeth rather than just 1 tooth.
- Teeth should be percussed in a random manner rather than the same order repeatedly.

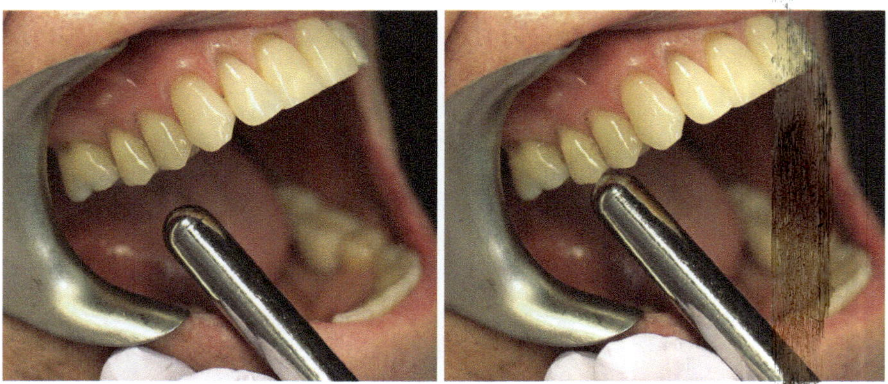

Fig. 3.13 Percussion using a mirror handle

Periodontal Probing

Periodontal probing may unexpectedly provide significant information. Deep periodontal defects may not be apparent on radiographs or visual examination. The defect may be due to a local problem or may be generalized or even be due to a root fracture. Information of this nature may alter the prognosis treatment plan of the case (Fig. 3.13).

Summary: Diagnostic Tests

Tests	Findings	Diagnosis	Treatment indicated
Cold	Severe or prolonged pain	Irreversible pulpitis	Root canal therapy or extraction
Heat	Pain	Devitalizing pulp	Root canal therapy or extraction
Palpation	Location of pain ex. Pain at apex, mid root, or at the gingival third	Based on location of sensitivity: root fracture, perforation, periodontal origin, or endodontic	Root canal therapy, extraction, periodontal treatment, or endodontics depending on diagnosis
Electric	Sensitivity	Vital pulp	None
	No sensitivity	Non-vital pulp or no response due to restoration	Possible root canal therapy, confirm with other tests cause of pain
Fiber optics (Transillumination)	Failure to transmit light through a tooth	Probable, vertical fracture	Further confirmation of fracture using a bite block, Tooth Sleuth©, and staining (methylene blue)
Bite block	Pain on biting or release of bite	Indication of probable fracture	Further confirmation of fracture using fiber optics, Tooth Sleuth©, and staining
Tooth Sleuth©	Pain on biting or release of bite	Indication of probable fracture	Further confirmation of fracture using fiber optics, Tooth Sleuth©, and staining

3.4 Additional Diagnostic Tool: Laser Doppler Flowmetry

Laser Doppler flowmetry has the ability to assess blood flow in the microvasculature, e.g., retina, mesentery, renal cortex, and skin. It has been shown to be able to detect blood circulation in human teeth [5]. Laser Doppler does not assess the degree of inflammatory changes in the pulp, and as with other pulp testing modalities, it has the risk of false positives and false negatives. The technique, although cumbersome, does have some important advantages. It is noninvasive and accurate in detecting revascularization of young traumatized teeth as confirmed by histologic observation in animal studies [5].

3.5 Tooth Fracture

Patients may present at an emergency visit with severe pain but without a clinically apparent cause. The patient may be able to localize the pain to a specific tooth, but the tooth may have only a shallow restoration or even be a virgin tooth. This mystery is often associated with a fracture that may be difficult to visualize. A good light source and magnification are important adjuncts to the diagnosis. Staining with methylene blue and use of a bite block are also useful in diagnosing a fracture.

The location, direction, and extent of a crack have a profound effect on the choice of treatment, so clarity of the diagnosis is important. Five types of longitudinal tooth fractures have been described as follows:

- Craze lines
- Split tooth
- Fractured cusp
- Vertical root fracture
- Cracked tooth

There are a number of factors and procedures helpful in identifying the presence of a crack.

- Dental history
- Periodontal probing
- Subjective examination
- Radiographic examination
- Objective visual examination
- Restoration removal
- Tactile examination
- Staining
- Periapical tests
- Transillumination
- Bite tests
- Wedging forces
- Vitality testing
- Surgical assessment

3.5.1 The History

As discussed in Chap. 1, listening to the history of the chief complaint is a critical part of diagnosing a fracture. It may enable the dentist to make a tentative diagnosis of a fracture even before examining the patient. Important questions are: "When did the pain start?" "What seemed to cause it?" "What relieves the pain?"

Often, patients with cracked teeth are able to describe a specific event that was followed immediately by a sharp pain. The event may be as simple as biting on a hard piece of popcorn or candy. At other times the event may be less dramatic but still marked the distinct starting point of pain. This scenario is a vital clue in the diagnosis of a fracture.

The American Association of Endodontists, *Colleagues for Excellence*, has published valuable material concerning the detection and treatment of various longitudinal tooth fractures. The issue titled, "Cracking the Cracked Tooth Code: Detection and Treatment of Various Longitudinal Tooth Fractures," is available online at www.aae.org/colleagues/.

3.5.2 Bite Block

Having a patient bite on a soft wood bite block is a classic technique for identifying a cracked tooth. A crack may not be visible clinically, and symptoms may be persistent without an obvious cause. Typically pain is elicited on release of the bite rather than on the application of pressure.

An alternative to a wooden bite stick is a Tooth Sleuth which is a plastic instrument designed to allow biting force to be isolated to a specific cusp or fossae of a tooth.

3.5.3 Transillumination

Craze lines are frequently confused with cracks but can be differentiated by transillumination. If the tooth has a through and through crack, the transmission of light will be blocked at the line of fracture, allowing only a segment of the tooth structure to light up. If the tooth has a craze line, the entire tooth will be illuminated.

Craze lines are thought to be points of weakness and have the potential to develop into cracks. It may be advantageous to restore teeth with craze lines with full coverage in an attempt to prevent progression of a craze line into a fracture.

3.5.4 Classic Signs of Cracked Teeth

Cracks in teeth often result in the so-called cracked tooth syndrome. The syndrome is characterized by acute pain on mastication (pressure or release) of grainy, tough foods and sharp, brief pain with cold. These findings are also related to cusp fracture.

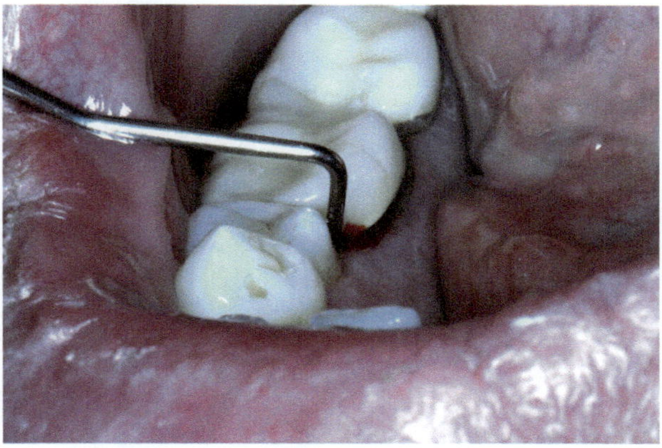

Fig. 3.14 Periodontal probing

Cracked teeth may present a variety of symptoms ranging from slight to severe spontaneous pain consistent with irreversible pulpitis, pulp necrosis, or apical periodontitis. Even an acute apical abscess, with or without swelling or a draining sinus tract, may be present if the pulp has undergone necrosis due to a crack. When a fracture has exposed the pulp, severe pulp and/or periapical pathosis follows. There may be significant variation in the signs and symptoms, associated with cracks (Figs. 3.14 and 3.15).

3.5.5 Craze Lines

Craze lines are thin, usually dark lines that appear to be superficial, without separation of adjacent segments. When examining teeth for cracks, it is important to understand that most adult teeth have craze lines. In posterior teeth, craze lines are usually evident crossing marginal ridges and extending along buccal and lingual surfaces. Long vertical craze lines also appear on anterior teeth. In some cases it may be difficult to differentiate a craze line from a fracture. Craze lines may represent a prelude to fracture, and no attempt should be made to wedge apart the segments on either side of the line.

Clinical Tips

- If endodontic therapy is initiated for a painful tooth, with craze lines, pain should disappear. Continued pain may indicate a fracture rather than a craze line. In such cases the probability of endodontic success is unlikely.

Treatment Planning for Teeth with Craze Lines

The significance of craze lines extending through the marginal ridge and into the floor of the chamber should be discussed with a patient. An analogy can be drawn between a craze line and similar lines seen in a dinner plate that remains in one piece but may fracture. Advising the patient of all reasonable options and documenting the findings can prevent problems in the future.

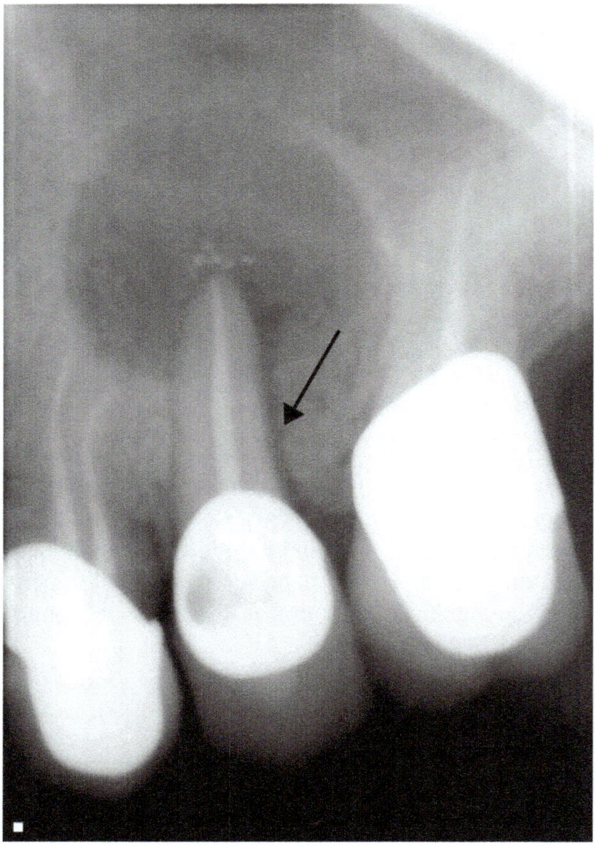

Fig. 3.15 Radiograph typical of a tooth with a vertical root fracture. *Arrow* points to a thickened periodontal membrane and periapical radiolucency typical of a vertical root fracture

Clinical Tips

- In cases where pain is eliminated after endodontic instrumentation, the use of full coverage may provide additional protection for the tooth.

References

1. American Association of Endodontists, American Academy of Oral and Maxillofacial Radiology (2011) Use of cone-beam computed tomography in endodontics Joint Position Statement of the American Association of Endodontists and the American Academy of Oral and Maxillofacial Radiology. Oral Surg Oral Med Oral Pathol Oral Radiol Endod 111(2):234–237
2. Carter L, Farman AG, Geist J et al (2008) American Academy of Oral and Maxillofacial Radiology executive opinion statement on performing and interpreting diagnostic cone beam computed tomography. Oral Surg Oral Med Oral Pathol Oral Radiol Endod 106(4):561–562
3. Cohenca N, Simon JH, Mathur A et al (2007) Clinical indications for digital imaging in dento-alveolar trauma. Part 2: root resorption. Dent Traumatol 23(2):105–113

4. Fulling HJ, Andreasen JO (1976) Influence of maturation status and tooth type of permanent teeth upon electrometric and thermal pulp testing. Scand J Dent Res 84(5):286–290
5. Hargreaves KM, Cohen S, Berman LH (2011) Cohen's pathways of the pulp. Mosby Elsevier, St. Louis
6. Hargreaves KM, Goodis HE (2012) Seltzer and Bender's dental pulp. Quintessence, Chicago
7. Hassan B, Metska ME, Ozok AR et al (2009) Detection of vertical root fractures in endodontically treated teeth by a cone beam computed tomography scan. J Endod 35(5):719–722
8. Hyman JJ, Cohen ME (1984) The predictive value of endodontic diagnostic tests. Oral Surg Oral Med Oral Pathol 58(3):343–346
9. Lofthag-Hansen S, Huumonen S, Grondahl K et al (2007) Limited cone-beam CT and intraoral radiography for the diagnosis of periapical pathology. Oral Surg Oral Med Oral Pathol Oral Radiol Endod 103(1):114–119
10. McCarthy PJ, McClanahan S, Hodges J et al (2010) Frequency of localization of the painful tooth by patients presenting for an endodontic emergency. J Endod 36(5):801–805
11. McGiff TJ, Danforth RA, Herschaft EE (2012) Maintaining radiation exposures as low as reasonably achievable (ALARA) for dental personnel operating portable hand-held x-ray equipment. Health Phys 103(2 Suppl 2):S179–S185
12. Petersson K, Soderstrom C, Kiani-Anaraki M et al (1999) Evaluation of the ability of thermal and electrical tests to register pulp vitality. Endod Dent Traumatol 15(3):127–131
13. Rosenberg PA, Frisbie J, Lee J et al (2010) Evaluation of pathologists (histopathology) and radiologists (cone beam computed tomography) differentiating radicular cysts from granulomas. J Endod 36(3):423–428

Pulpal and Periapical Diagnostic Terminology and Treatment Considerations

4

4.1 Synthesis of Information

The final pulpal and periapical diagnosis is based on a synthesis of information collected from the patient's history of the chief complaint, dental and medical histories, radiographs, sensibility, and clinical tests. The process is challenging since no single test can be considered definitive.

The clinician should have a keen ear capable of interpreting subtle clues in the patient's narrative and be able to put the clues together with other diagnostic information. At the same time, the clinician must recognize false leads that can result in misdiagnosis and treating the wrong tooth or providing treatment that is not necessary. Tests provide information, but the critical part of the diagnostic process is the ability of the clinician to synthesize information into a rational meaningful complete picture.

4.2 Terminology

There is more than one set of terms used to describe pulp and periapical pathosis. Terminology varies among different organizations to describe the pulp and periapical tissues. Variation in terminology can cause confusion during communication with other dentists (as can different dental numbering systems).

It must be understood that inflamed pulp tissue is in a dynamic state and may have more than one condition existing in the tissue at the same time. For example, underlying deep caries there may be an area of acute inflammation adjacent to chronic inflammation and/or necrosis all of which is in flux. These states may coexist asymptomatically for a long period of time or degenerate rapidly to total necrosis with or without pain. It has been clearly demonstrated that clinical symptoms do not correlate well with histologic findings [7, 9].

The dynamic state of the tissue can produce confusing results during sensibility testing. For example, a root canal may contain necrotic tissue but still have some neural tissue capable of conducting an impulse. In such cases a positive response to

P.A. Rosenberg, *Endodontic Pain*,
DOI 10.1007/978-3-642-54701-0_4, © Springer-Verlag Berlin Heidelberg 2014

testing with cold or electric could mislead the clinician into a diagnosis of a normal responsive pulp. Similarly in a multi-rooted tooth, one root may contain responsive pulp tissue, while the other is completely necrotic. In that case, pulp testing would not indicate the presence of pulp necrosis.

The American Association of Endodontists (AAE) recently published (2012) a revised list of pulp and periapical diagnostic terms and definitions (Table 4.1). The terminology is useful in categorizing cases and their treatment. There are other pulp classifications, but the AAE provides the most recent revision available. There is no universal agreement concerning the validity of this terminology.

4.3 Neuroplasticity

A major development in the field of pain physiology was the discovery of neuroplasticity in the late twentieth century. According to this concept, experiences like thinking, learning, and habits (addiction) can significantly change both the brain's physical structure (anatomy) and its functional organization (physiology). Neuroplasticity has an obvious positive side, including all forms of learning and adaptive responses to injury or other personal experiences. However, it also can have a destructive effect due to negative experiences [3].

Neuroplasticity may explain expanded areas of patients' perception of pain beyond what might be expected (i.e., the area of the body feeling pain is more extensive than that which was actually injured) or as chronic pain (i.e., the original injury or disease has resolved, but the pain remains and may even increase). Both of these are examples of a negative manifestation of neuroplasticity, which explains many previously misunderstood phenomena but also poses a significant management challenge for pain therapists and dentists. All dentists and physicians should appreciate the implications of neuroplasticity since it helps understanding their patients' complaints of pain [3].

"Neuroplasticity" is a term that describes how the nervous system changes in response to painful and other stimuli. To understand this process, it is important to recognize that the simple model of a painful stimulus leading to a proportional response has been replaced by a much more complex model of nervous system behavior.

The following sections will amplify each of the diagnostic terms.

4.4 Reversible Pulpitis

This highly subjective term is based on the history of the chief complaint as well as information drawn from radiographs and sensibility tests. A reversible pulpitis must be seen in the context of tissue in a dynamic state. There is no single diagnostic test that provides defining data about the exact histologic state of the pulp or its prognosis.

Table 4.1 A 2012 revision of terminology by the American Association of Endodontists indicates both the previous and most current terms and definitions

Old term	New term	Definition
Normal pulp	Normal pulp	A clinical diagnostic category in which the pulp is symptom-free and normally responsive to pulp testing
Reversible pulpitis	Reversible pulpitis	A clinical diagnosis based upon subjective and objective findings indicating that the inflammation should resolve and the pulp return to normal
Irreversible pulpitis	Symptomatic irreversible pulpitis	A clinical diagnosis based on subjective and objective findings indicating that the vital inflamed pulp is incapable of healing. *Additional descriptors*: lingering thermal pain, spontaneous pain, referred pain
	Asymptomatic irreversible pulpitis	A clinical diagnosis based on subjective and objective findings indicating that the vital inflamed pulp is incapable of healing. *Additional descriptors:* no clinical symptoms but inflammation produced by caries, caries excavation, trauma, etc.
Pulp necrosis	Pulp necrosis	A clinical diagnostic category indicating death of the dental pulp. The pulp is usually nonresponsive to pulp testing
Previously treated (pulpless)	Previously treated	A clinical diagnostic category indicating that the tooth has been endodontically treated and the canals are obturated with various filling materials other than intra-canal medicaments
Normal periapical (periradicular) tissues	Normal apical tissues	Teeth with normal periradicular tissues that is not sensitive to percussion or palpation testing. The lamina dura surrounding the root is intact, and the periodontal ligament space is uniform
Acute periapical (periradicular) periodontitis or chronic apical (periradicular) periodontitis with symptoms	Symptomatic apical periodontitis	Inflammation, usually of the apical periodontium, producing clinical symptoms including a painful response to biting and/or percussion or palpation. It may or may not be associated with an apical radiolucent area
Chronic periapical (periradicular) abscess periodontitis	Asymptomatic apical periodontitis	Inflammation and destruction of apical periodontium that is of pulpal origin appears as an apical radiolucent area and does not produce clinical symptoms

(continued)

Table 4.1 (continued)

Old term	New term	Definition
Acute apical (periradicular) abscess	Acute apical abscess	An inflammatory reaction to pulpal infection and necrosis characterized by rapid onset, spontaneous pain, extreme tenderness of the tooth to pressure, pus formation, and swelling of associated tissues
Chronic apical (periradicular) abscess or phoenix abscess or suppurative apical periodontitis	Chronic apical abscess	An inflammatory reaction to pulpal infection and necrosis characterized by gradual onset, little or no discomfort, and the intermittent discharge of pus through an associated sinus tract
Focal sclerosing osteomyelitis	Condensing osteitis	Diffuse radiopaque lesion representing a localized bony reaction to a low-grade inflammatory stimulus, usually seen at apex of the tooth

American Association of Endodontists and the American Board of Endodontics Terminology (2012)

The American Association of Endodontists publishes a newsletter, *Endodontics Colleagues for Excellence*, and the Fall 2013 edition is titled Endodontic Diagnosis. Included in that issue is a description of current diagnostic terminology and self-assessment sample cases. The newsletters can be accessed at www.aae.org/colleagues/.

The clinician must synthesize all available data including history of the pain, its severity, and the treatment plan. The patient's narrative is extremely important.

Important questions for the patient include:

- *When did the pain start?*
- *Did it follow a new restoration or occur spontaneously?*
- *What makes the tooth hurt?*
- *What makes the pain stop?*
- *Did the pain start suddenly after biting on something hard?*
- *Is the pain getting worse?*
- *Does it wake you up at night?*
- *Can you chew on the tooth without pain?*
- *What medication are you using for pain? Is it effective?*
- *On a scale of 1–10 with 1 being very mild and 10 being unbearable, how would you rank your pain?*

Radiographic findings may include the presence of decay, old pulp caps, large restorations, periodontal disease, all of which add to the picture. The patient's response to the above questions, combined with diagnostic findings point the way to determining if the diagnosis is of odontogenic or non-odontogenic origin. It helps to clarify if there is reversible pulpitis, not requiring intervention, or requires treatment.

The clinician should explain his diagnosis and treatment plan to the patient and note that additional follow-up may be required.

4.5 Cold Sensitivity Following a Restorative Procedure

A complaint of cold sensitivity after an operative procedure requires follow-up to determine if the symptom of cold sensitivity disappears, remains the same, or gets worse over days, weeks, or months. A particularly difficult question occurs when there is a persistent moderate level of pain that neither progresses toward less pain nor does not increase in severity. Clearly, there is a time period beyond which it is not reasonable to wait any longer to make a decision about treatment from patient to patient. There is no simple answer to the question of how long to wait, and the variables include patient's dental history, severity of pain, and the ultimate treatment plan.

For example, if the tooth in question is to be restored with a crown, there should be no question about the status of the pulp when the restoration is completed and ready to be cemented. If moderate pain persists over a number of weeks or there is an inability to use the tooth during function, it becomes increasingly clear that endodontic therapy is necessary.

At no time should the patient be pushed into treatment that he/she does not fully understand or desire. In cases where there is severe pain that suddenly disappears, it is advisable to apply sensibility tests again in order to determine if the absence of pain is due to healing or devitalization.

Clinical Tips

- Do not place a final restoration until the status of the pulp is resolved.
- Root canal therapy cannot "always be done later," without damaging the restoration. For example, consider the difference between treating a mandibular incisor with or without a crown present. The narrowness of the prepared tooth under the crown would make access difficult and probably result in damage to the integrity of the crown.

4.6 Symptomatic Irreversible Pulpitis

This diagnosis is based on subjective and objective findings that lead to a conclusion that the pulp in question does not have the capacity to heal. Important factors to consider include the presumed cause of the pain, its severity and duration, as well as the patient's ability to use it during function.

For example, a large pulp exposure due to caries or a traumatic fracture represents serious problems that would not be considered reversible. In contrast, pain sensitivity following a crown preparation may not be immediately recognized as reversible or irreversible. Severe lingering pain after the application of cold or heat sensitivity is taken as a classic sign of irreversible pulpitis. Irreversible pulpitis can be treated by endodontic therapy or extraction.

Clinical Tips

When treating a tooth with irreversible pulpitis:

- Teeth with irreversible pulpitis often pose a challenge in achieving complete dental anesthesia. It is beneficial to test a tooth with cold, heat, or percussion (the chief complaint) rather than just depending on a numb lip to be an indicator of successful anesthesia.
- Be prepared to utilize alternative anesthetic techniques including intraosseous, ligamental, and intrapulpal injections.
- If time does not permit complete instrumentation of a canal(s), pulpotomy (all tissue from the chamber is removed but canal(s) is not entered) has been shown to be an effective means of reducing pain.
- Following measurement control, all pulp tissue should be removed from the canal(s). Never partially instrument a canal. Leaving shredded pulp tissue behind can cause increased pain.
- If there is concomitant sensitivity to percussion, the occlusion should be relieved unless contraindicated by restorative issues.

4.7 Pulp Necrosis

Necrosis is an end stage of pulp inflammation and represents death of the pulp. There is no longer a functioning circulatory system nor are there responsive nerve fibers present. The pulp no longer has the capacity for repair. Swelling may be associated with pulp necrosis if the pathogenic process extends into the periapical tissues. Pulp testing elicits no response regardless of the modality used. Treatment for pulp necrosis is either endodontic therapy or extraction.

Treatment of a tooth with a necrotic pulp poses a microbiological challenge because the canal system is infected with a mix of anaerobic and aerobic bacteria. It is extremely important to instrument, irrigate, and fill a canal while not pushing contaminated debris through the periapical foramina into the surrounding tissue.

A necrotic pulp may be associated with an asymptomatic or severely painful tooth. There may or may not be a periapical lesion present on radiographs, and sensibility tests would not elicit a response. Depending on the thickness of the bone, palpation may or may not induce pain. In the asymptomatic tooth without a periapical lesion, the diagnosis of pulp necrosis is best verified by a negative response to heat, cold, and electric testing. Adjacent teeth must also be tested.

Clinical Tips

- In some cases large restorations or pulp calcification can interfere with the transmission of provoking stimuli. This may cause a clinician to misdiagnose a tooth and inadvertently initiate treatment on a tooth that has a vital pulp.
- Never partially instrument a canal. When a canal is entered, its contents must be completely removed.
- Irrigation with sodium hypochlorite (NaOCl) is a critical part of instrumentation due to its potent bacteriocidal activity and tissue dissolving capability.

4.8 Previously Treated Teeth

This category includes teeth with failed previously completed root canal therapy. The endodontic failure may be associated with pain/swelling, or a periapical lesion that did not respond to treatment, or a new lesion that did not exist prior to endodontic treatment. It has been amply demonstrated that bacteria play the primary role in endodontic failures (Fig. 4.1) [4].

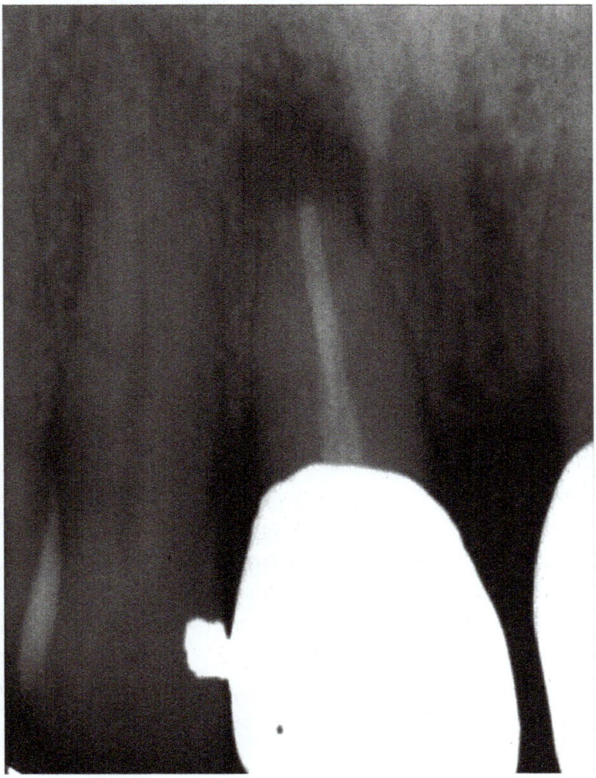

Fig. 4.1 Failing root canal therapy. Following emergency treatment, the case will be retreated and followed to determine if apical surgery is required. *Footnote*: This radiograph demonstrates previously treated tooth #8. Please note the periapical lesion and apical resorption. The patient presented in severe pain, without swelling, isolated to #8. Following emergency treatment, non-surgical root canal therapy will be redone. The patient will be followed to determine the need for apical surgery

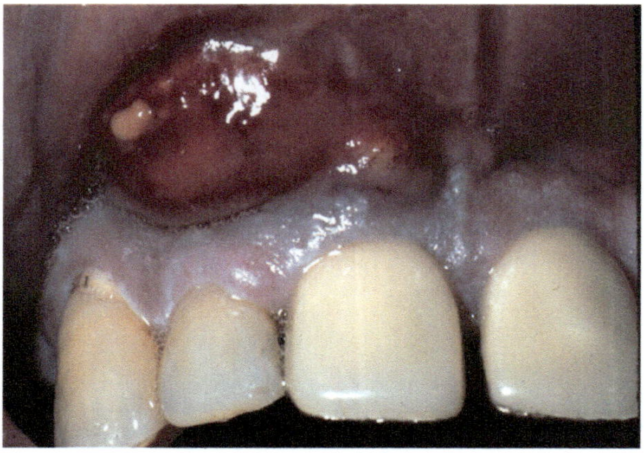

Fig. 4.2 Circumscribed swelling associated with failing root canal therapy. At the emergency visit the prior root canal filling should be removed. Cleaning/shaping with NaOCl irrigation is appropriate. A $CaOH_2$ dressing is placed in the canal. Incision and drainage is indicated due to the fluctuant nature of the swelling

Previously treated teeth present challenges not always associated with initial endodontic treatment. The differences start at the treatment planning stage when the clinician must determine if nonsurgical retreatment, surgical treatment, or a combination offers the best prognosis [1, 2, 6].

There may be obstacles to nonsurgical retreatment in terms of posts or restorative concerns. The clinician must determine if a post can be removed and if that will cause significant weakening of the tooth, resulting in fracture. These factors might tilt the treatment plan toward a surgical approach.

Presence of new crowns or laminates is also a factor to consider. If retreatment is likely to seriously damage the restoration, it may be best to consider a surgical approach depending on the quality of the initial treatment. If the initial endodontic treatment is clearly deficient, it reduces the prognosis of surgical therapy without retreatment. This decision must be made on a case-by-case basis (Figs. 4.1 and 4.2).

Questions to consider when assessing a previously treated case:

- *Are residual bacteria in the root canal system due to inadequate endodontic treatment or due to an inadequate restoration that may have to be replaced?*
- *Is nonsurgical retreatment feasible, or are there restorative obstacles?*
- *If there is a post present, can it be removed without destroying excessive tooth structure?*
- *Is there a poor crown to root ratio?*
- *Has a fracture been ruled out?*
- *After endodontic retreatment will there be enough tooth structure left to restore?*
- *Is there a periodontal lesion present that may have contributed to the failure?*
- *Is the plan cost-effective and the prognosis good, or would an implant be a better alternative?*

The answers to these questions help to determine the prognosis of retreatment with or without surgery. Meticulous retrospective studies concluded that the estimated success rate of secondary root canal treatment was 77 %. The presence of a preoperative periapical lesion, periapical extent of root filling, and quality of coronal restoration proved significant prognostic factors [6].

The economics of retreatment or extraction and implant is another important consideration. The cost and prognosis of retreatment must be weighed against the cost of an implant to replace the tooth. All reasonable treatment plan options must be presented to the patient who ultimately makes the final decision [4].

4.9 Symptomatic Periapical Periodontitis

Symptomatic periapical periodontitis can cause pain ranging from minor to so severe that even tongue pressure can elicit severe pain. It may or may not be associated with a periapical radiolucent area [8]. It often represents an extension of pulp pathosis into the periodontium. If excess occlusion due to a new restoration, or a fracture, or an acute periodontal lesion can be ruled out, the likely cause of the pain is an extension of pulp pathosis into the periodontal ligament.

4.10 Asymptomatic Periapical Periodontitis

In cases where inflammation and destruction of the periapical periodontium is of pulpal origin, a periapical radiolucent area may be present. It may or may not be associated with symptoms. A necrotic pulp, due to the presence of microbes, results in immune and inflammatory reactions in the periapical tissue. Ultimately, those reactions release mediators associated with bone resorption and radiographic radiolucency.

It is important to note that asymptomatic periodontitis may revert to an acute or chronic periapical abscess with or without severe pain. This is a dynamic situation and alterations in the virulence and/or numbers of microbes or diminished host resistance can result in the clinical symptoms.

Asymptomatic periapical periodontitis represents pathosis that requires either root canal therapy or extraction. The lesion has the potential to form an abscess, granuloma, or periapical cyst without a change in the clinical symptoms. Precise determination of the lesion can be accomplished only by biopsy and not just by radiographs.

4.11 Chronic Periapical Abscess

A chronic periapical abscess is an inflammatory reaction to pulpal infection and necrosis characterized by gradual onset, little or no discomfort, and often the intermittent discharge of pus through an associated sinus. Due to the lack of symptoms, this lesion is often discovered on radiographic examination. It is not unusual to find an extensive radiolucency that has not caused pain. Diagnosis of chronic periapical abscess should be confirmed with sensibility tests. A vital response to thermal or electric tests should be recognized as a warning that the cause may be non-odontogenic.

When a clinical examination identifies a stoma, it must be traced. Typically a gutta-percha cone is gently threaded into the stoma and may indicate that its origin

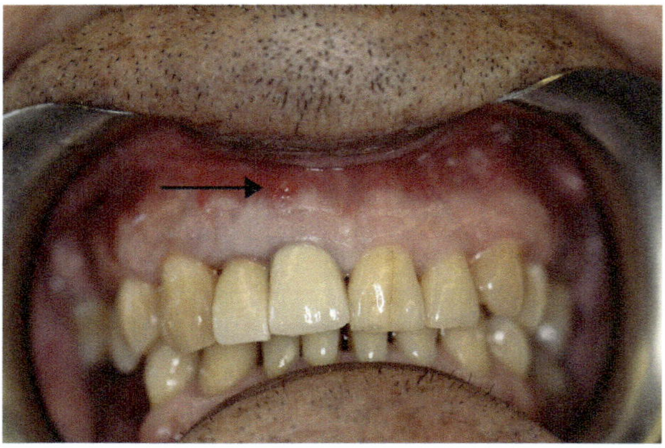

Fig. 4.3 *Arrow* points to stoma present in the mucobuccal fold

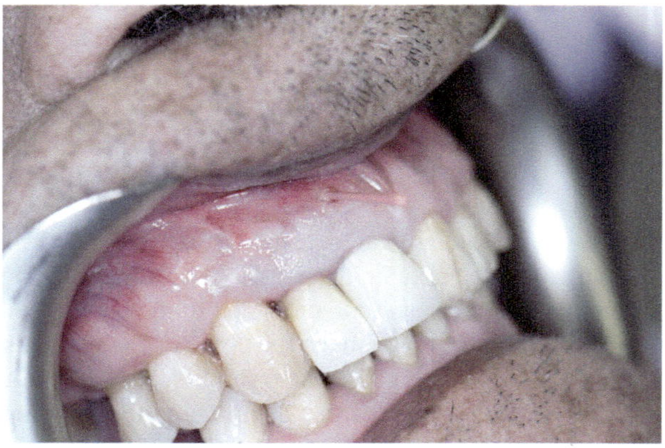

Fig. 4.4 Gutta-percha cone inserted into stoma

is some distance from the closest tooth. Treatment is either endodontic therapy or extraction. A chronic periapical abscess cannot heal without endodontic intervention (Figs 4.3, 4.4, and 4.5).

4.12 Acute Periapical Abscess

An acute periapical abscess is a localized inflammatory reaction to pulpal infection and necrosis. It is characterized by rapid onset, spontaneous pain, tenderness to pressure, pus formation, and swelling. Untreated, it may progress to poorly localized cellulitis. Patients with this condition are often seen at an emergency visit due to severe pain and swelling. Radiographic findings vary. Radiographic findings vary from extensive lesions to only thickening of the periodontal membrane.

Treatment is focused on canal cleaning/shaping and irrigation with sodium hypochlorite. This approach is directed at reducing the bacterial content in the root canal system that is the ultimate cause of the problem. Incision and drainage may be performed selectively in cases with fluctuant swellings. Incision and drainage of an

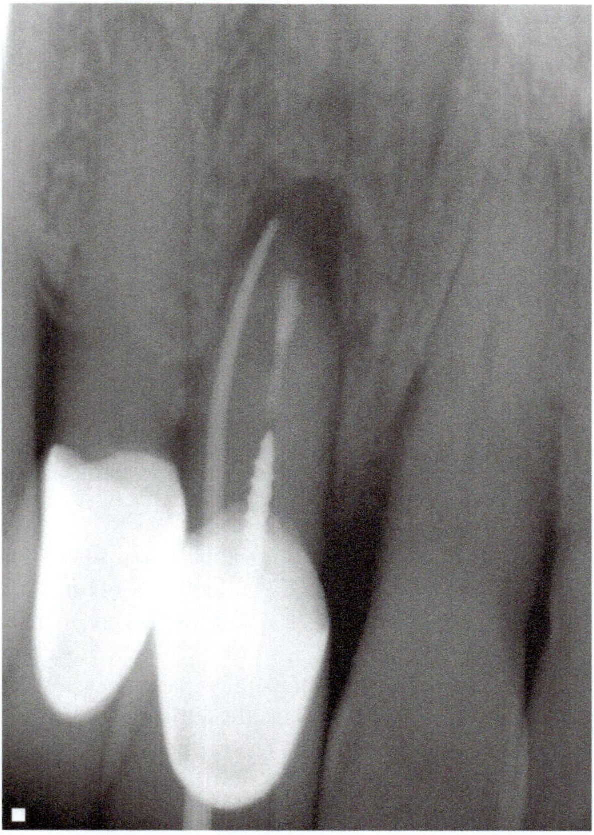

Fig. 4.5 Radiograph of gutta-percha cone tracing sinus tract

abscess may reduce pain by reducing concentrations of bacterial toxins and mediators as well as by lowering tissue pressure.

Diffuse, poorly localized lesions with extensive swelling, presence of fever, and systemic comorbidities indicate the need for a supplementary antibiotic as a secondary line of defense.

During treatment of abscessed teeth, it is advisable to have the patient return frequently for re-cleaning/shaping and irrigation even after the patient has been placed on antibiotic therapy. The goal is to eliminate resistant microbes and tissue remnants from the canal space (Fig. 4.6).

4.13 Hospitalization of Patients with Dental Abscesses

Investigators conducted a retrospective analysis of patients admitted to hospitals with a primary diagnosis of periapical abscess between 2000 and 2008. Patient characteristics analyzed included age, sex, race, presence of comorbid conditions, and insurance status.

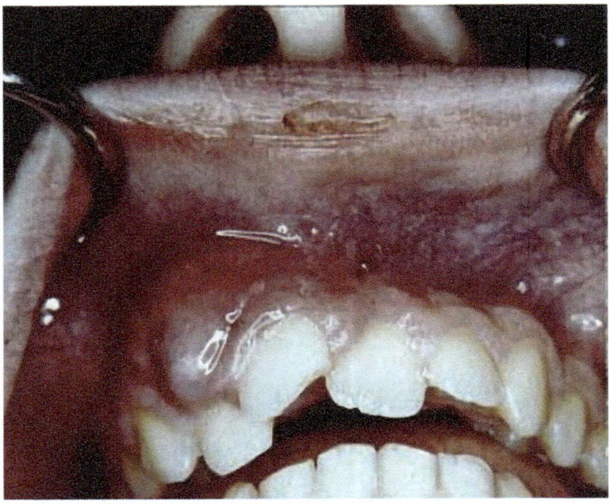

Fig. 4.6 Well-defined circumscribed swelling. Sensibility test will be required to identify the cause of the problem

During the 9-year period, the number of people admitted for dental abscesses rose significantly from 5,757 in 2000 to 8,141 in 2008.

This represents a 41.4 % increase in hospitalizations of patients with dental abscesses.

In addition, a total of 61,439 patients were admitted for dental infections. The number of in-hospital deaths attributed to the infections was 66.

Admissions occurred on an emergency basis in 89 % of those hospitalized, and the mean length of hospital stay was nearly 3 days. Patients with sinus involvement stayed longer in the hospital as did older patients. The average patient age was 37 years.

A number of socioeconomic, demographic, and therapeutic factors may be involved in these findings. Economic pressures and insurance issues may keep patients from seeking preventive dental treatment and impact on their access to care [10].

4.13.1 Cellulitis

As in all infected cases, debridement of the canal(s), and irrigation followed by placement of calcium hydroxide, is the basic treatment for a patient presenting with diffuse facial swelling (cellulitis) resulting from an acute apical abscess. Systemic involvement in the form of fever or malaise may also be noted (Fig. 4.7).

This situation is different than the patient presenting with a well-localized swelling although the basic cause remains bacterial invasion of the root canal system and an apical reaction. However, in the case of cellulitis, the host's defensive systems

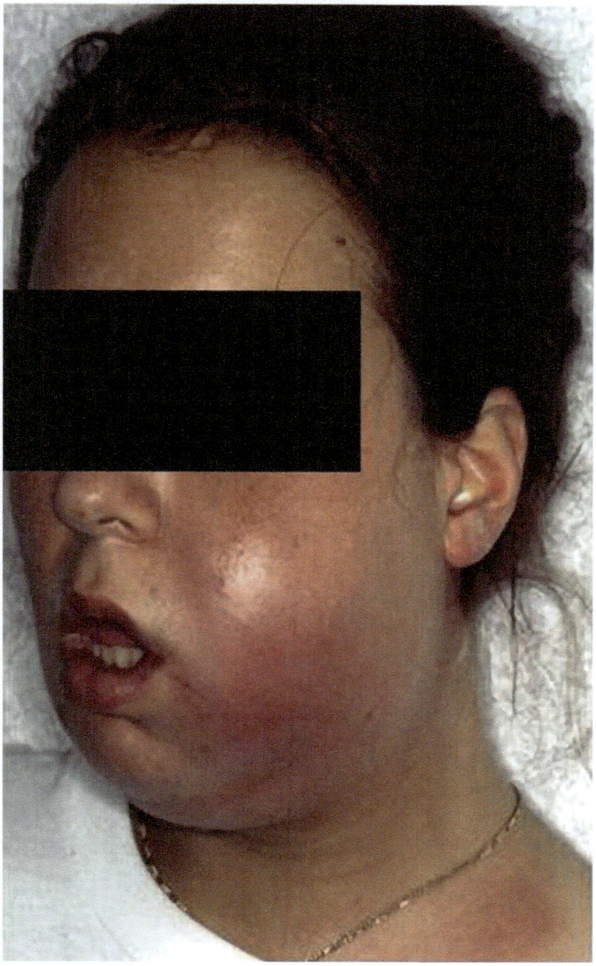

Fig. 4.7 Cellulitis extending into the buccinators and submandibular spaces

have been unable to achieve localization and limit the spread of the pathogenic process. Due to the lack of localization, there is a more serious potential associated with a cellulitis in contrast to an abscess. A patient with a cellulitis must be monitored closely and is more likely to be given an antibiotic than a patient treated for a well-localized abscess. Some cellulitis patients, especially those with complex medical histories, may require hospitalization and intravenous administration of an antibiotic.

Despite the different presentation of an abscess and cellulitis, bacterial causation remains the same. Treatment must be directed at eliminating bacteria from the canal space. Frequent cleaning/shaping and irrigation remain the key procedures directed at reducing the bacterial content of the canal system.

Surgical incision for drainage in cases of cellulitis may not be productive. The mucobuccal tissues may appear almost normal because the exudate has migrated through facial planes beyond the confines of the apical tissues. In such cases a regimen of systemic antibiotics, cleaning/shaping, and irrigation is appropriate.

Clinical Tips

- Drainage from canals will usually stop shortly after instrumentation allowing placement of calcium hydroxide and closure of the tooth.
- During the treatment of abscesses or of cellulitis, the teeth should be closed between visits.
- Leaving the teeth open between visits permits further ingress of bacteria into the canal system. This is counterproductive to the treatment goal of eliminating bacteria from the canal system.

4.14 Persistent Stomas

In some cases despite repeated cleaning/shaping and irrigation, a stoma will persist. In some cases, after completion of a nonsurgical or surgical case, a stoma may reappear after a short time. There are several possibilities in such situations. It is important to resist the temptation to use antibiotic therapy in these cases. Although the stoma may close temporarily, the biological cause of the problem has not been identified.

4.14.1 Common Causes of Persistent Stomas

- Periodontal complication.
- Fractured root.
- The incorrect tooth was treated.
- Extra-radicular infection.

4.15 Condensing Osteitis

Condensing osteitis is viewed as a diffuse radiopaque lesion representing a localized bony reaction to a low-grade inflammatory stimulus, usually seen at apex of a tooth. This lesion has also been called focal sclerosing osteomyelitis.

It may be associated with previous pulp caps or deep restorations causing chronic pulp inflammation with or without intermittent pulpal symptoms. The chronic nature of the inflammatory lesion may sensitize the pulp and interfere with successful pulpal anesthesia (Fig. 4.8).

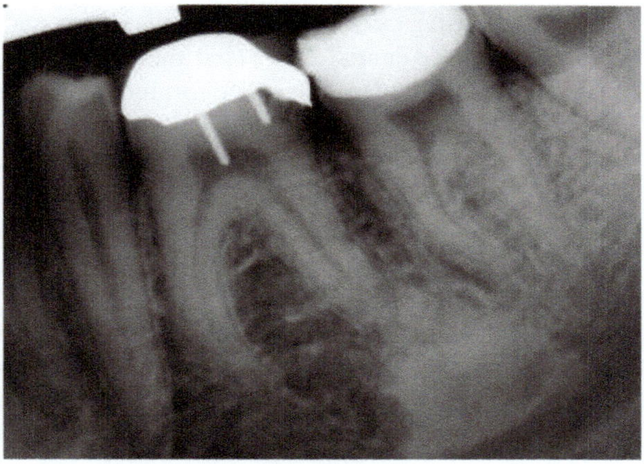

Fig. 4.8 Chronic inflammation, over a long period of time, can cause sclerotic lesions as seen in this image. The long-standing inflammation can also result in a tooth that is difficult to anesthetize due to changes in nociceptors

Clinical Tips

- Radiographic repair of sclerotic lesions has been reported, but it usually takes much longer than healing of radiolucent lesions.
- Careful diagnostic questioning of a patient with a periapical sclerotic lesion often produces a narrative that includes intermittent low-level pain and difficulty masticating.
- Sensibility test results may vary but often include thermal sensitivity.
- Elimination of symptoms requires endodontic therapy.
- Profound local anesthesia may be difficult to achieve due to a history of chronic inflammation and sensitivity of nociceptors (pain receptors).
- Supplemental anesthetic techniques are often necessary.

4.16 Atypical Odontalgia: An Oral Neuropathic Pain Phenomenon

4.16.1 A Classic Description of a Patient with Atypical Odontalgia

A new patient visited a dentist with a history of pain for 10 months duration. The patient described the pain as originating from the posterior left mandibular quadrant. The pain was not associated with mastication, and there was no sensitivity to heat or cold stimuli. Percussion of the teeth in the maxillary and mandibular quadrants was unproductive.

Previous treatment directed at resolving the problem included endodontic treatment for the mandibular left first premolar that was unsuccessful. The patient, a woman, was caries-free and had only small occlusal restorations in the quadrant.

After extensive examination of the maxillary and mandibular posterior quadrants, her former dentist diagnosed the problem as irreversible pulpitis of the left mandibular first premolar. The former dentist initiated endodontic treatment for that tooth, and cleaning/shaping and irrigation resulted in relief of pain for several days. However, the pain returned several days later. Obturation of the canals resulted in no significant change. The patient became convinced that the pain was now coming from the mandibular left first molar, so the new dentist agreed to explore that tooth, leading to another unsuccessful endodontic treatment.

An endodontist was consulted and he retreated both teeth and performed apical surgery on the mesial root of the first molar, but no improvement resulted. The patient became convinced that the pain was now emanating from other teeth in the region, and she was angry with her previous dentists for not resolving this problem.

This classic case was resolved after the endodontist referred the patient to an orofacial pain specialist for appropriate medical management of her chronic pain. Management of this problem is best accomplished by orofacial pain experts who have formal training, as well as by neurologists and other pain management physicians.

It is likely that this phenomenon is an example of a certain type of neuropathic pain that in the past has been labeled with such names as "phantom tooth pain" and "atypical facial pain." However, in recent years this phenomenon most widely has been called "atypical odontalgia" (AO).

Following is a brief review of neuropathic pain in order to provide better understanding of this phenomenon. It is followed by a discussion of AO, with special emphasis on how the treatment of these patients may be managed in a dental office. Early recognition of the diagnosis is the key to avoiding the scenario in the case described above.

4.16.2 Overview of Neuropathic Pain

A noxious stimulus to any peripheral structure activates nociceptors or pain receptors, producing nerve impulses that travel to the brain for the perception of pain. This acute pain often is termed "nociceptive pain" because it arises from the direct activation of nociceptors.

Neuropathic pain, on the other hand, is pain arising as a result of a lesion or disease affecting the actual nerves that convey information about touch, pressure, pain, and temperature from the body (skin, muscles, joints, bone) to the brain [11]. In some cases, neuropathic pain can arise spontaneously, for reasons that are not yet understood.

Atypical Odontalgia: Changing Terminology

The term, "atypical odontalgia," is being revised by the Orofacial Pain Special Interest Group of the International Association for the Study of Pain. The new term, which is more specific, will be "chronic continuous dentoalveolar pain" (CCDAP).

The diagnostic criteria for this condition are:

- Chronic continuous pain
- Pain localized in the dentoalveolar region
- Pain not caused by another disorder

This change from "atypical odontalgia" (AO) to "chronic continuous dentoalveolar pain" (CCDAP) is part of a major overhaul of terminology in the orofacial pain field that should lead to an improved diagnostic taxonomy.

Warning
It is important that dentists avoid being drawn into performing multiple dental procedures when confronted with situations that are similar to the one previously described. Such patients are often convinced that their pain is localized in a tooth or teeth.

When the patient's description of pain and its origin cannot be substantiated by clinical examination and sensibility tests, it represents a critical warning sign for the dentist. It is important to remember that repeated procedures in the painful region not only will fail to produce relief and may result in increased pain following each intervention.

Patients who appear to have this type of problem should be told that they must see an orofacial pain expert—preferably sooner rather than later. If the diagnosis proves to be neuropathic pain, both the patient and the dentist will be glad that unnecessary and expensive dental treatment was avoided.

4.17 Self-Assessment

- How do I proceed if I cannot determine if pain is originating in the maxillae or mandible?

  An inferior mandibular block injection can be helpful in determining the origin of pain. If pain persists after local anesthesia, it is likely that the offending tooth is in the maxillary arch or it is of non-odontogenic origin. If pain disappears after the block injection, it is a reasonable assumption that pain stems from a mandibular tooth (odontogenic origin).
- How do I differentiate odontogenic pain from temporomandibular pain?

  Typically patients with TMD have a chronic history of the problem. Palpation of the intraoral and extraoral musculature may reveal muscular tenderness.

  Limited ability to open the mouth wide and/or deviation to one side may indicate muscular or joint dysfunction.
- How do I differentiate atypical facial pain or headache pain from endodontic pain?

  The patient's dental history and chief complaint are important. Atypical facial pain or headache pain usually has a long history. There is often an absence of specific dental complaints. There may be no history of thermal sensitivity or of an inability to eat using the tooth or teeth in question. Clinical and sensibility tests are normal in patients with atypical facial pain or headache pain. Absence of specific dental symptoms is an important clue.

- A patient presents with a chief complaint of sensitivity to cold and identifies the mandibular right first molar as the site of pain. The patient's pain is not severe. You are unable to reproduce the symptom despite using several test modalities. Other tests, including percussion and palpation, are unproductive.

  The patient urges you to provide treatment for the suspect tooth because he is a busy person and does not want to waste time on another visit. What is your treatment plan?

  Defer treatment until diagnostic tests substantiate the patient's impression. Multiple tests are important, as are radiographs from different angles. The patient should be monitored carefully.

Clinical Tips

There are often clues in the patient's history that signal the possibility of non-odontogenic pain.

The following clues may indicate a non-odontogenic cause of pain:

A history that does not include:

- Thermal sensitivity
- An inability to use the suspect tooth or teeth during mastication
- Words like tingling or burning to describe the pain

Additional clues suggesting non-odontogenic pain:

- A lack of a painful response to the normal pain-provoking diagnostic stimuli
- Previous root canal treatment for other teeth, in the same area, to address the same complaint
- A long history of the same complaint over months or years
- Presence of other chronic pain conditions including temporomandibular joint dysfunction, chronic headaches, or neuralgia [5]
- Several missing teeth in the same area
- A history of previous endodontic treatment followed by extraction
- A muscle trigger point for pain
- Limited intermaxillary opening or deviation from the midline on opening

A new patient comes to your dental office with severe pain in the upper left quadrant. The patient has experienced a dull aching pain in the upper left first molar for 3 weeks. The history of the chief complaint, clinical examination, and sensibility tests validate that the pain is coming from the maxillary left first molar.

The pain is worse in the morning, upon awakening, and then dissipates during the day. Examination reveals that endodontic treatment had been performed 2 years earlier for that tooth. There is no sensitivity to percussion, and radiographs demonstrate endodontic treatment with well-filled canals. No clinical or radiographic evidence of disease is associated with the maxillary left first molar.

On palpation of the musculature, the masseter muscle is extremely tender. The patient is able to eat comfortably, and there is no thermal sensitivity in the area.

What is the most likely explanation for these observations, and what would your treatment plan be for this patient?

The history and symptoms described are consistent with a diagnosis of referred pain. Referred pain (synonymous with heterotopic pain) is felt at a site distant from the site of origin and frequently is found in patients with chronic musculoskeletal pain (e.g., temporomandibular disorders, fibromyalgia, low back pain).

Although superficial pain (e.g., that from a denture-induced ulcer or a periapical abscess) is usually is sharp, intense, and well localized, it is rarely referred. Muscle pain is a deep pain that usually is dull, aching, cramping, and difficult to localize. Often, it is referred to other structures such as the temporomandibular joint and teeth.

The mechanisms involved in acute superficial pain are well known, and dental and medical clinicians are skilled in its management. Less information is available about the mechanisms involved in muscle pain and, in particular, how such pain arises. As a consequence, muscle pain usually is much more difficult to manage.

4.17.1 Treatment Plan

It is important to note that pain that is worse in the morning and dissipates during the day. This is usually associated with musculature or joint dysfunction, and treatment should be directed toward that area. There is no indication for endodontic treatment in this case.

References

1. Friedman S, Stabholz A (1986) Endodontic retreatment–case selection and technique. Part 1: criteria for case selection. J Endod 12(1):28–33
2. Friedman S, Stabholz A, Tamse A (1990) Endodontic retreatment–case selection and technique. 3. Retreatment techniques. J Endod 16(11):543–549
3. Greene CS (2009) Neuroplasticity and sensitization. J Am Dent Assoc 140(6):676–678
4. Hargreaves KM, Cohen S, Berman LH (2011) Cohen's pathways of the pulp. Mosby Elsevier, St. Louis
5. Murray GM (2009) Referred pain, allodynia and hyperalgesia. J Am Dent Assoc 140(9):1122–1124
6. Ng YL, Mann V, Gulabivala K (2008) Outcome of secondary root canal treatment: a systematic review of the literature. Int Endod J 41(12):1026–1046
7. Peters DD, Baumgartner JC, Lorton L (1994) Adult pulpal diagnosis. I. Evaluation of the positive and negative responses to cold and electrical pulp tests. J Endod 20(10):506–511
8. Rosenberg PA, Schindler WG, Krell KV et al (2009) Identify the endodontic treatment modalities. J Endod 35(12):1675–1694

9. Seltzer S, Bender IB, Ziontz M (1963) The dynamics of pulp inflammation: correlations between diagnostic data and actual histologic findings in the pulp. Oral Surg Oral Med Oral Pathol 16:969–977
10. Shah AC, Leong KK, Lee MK et al (2013) Outcomes of hospitalizations attributed to periapical abscess from 2000 to 2008: a longitudinal trend analysis. J Endod 39(9):1104–1110
11. Treede RD, Jensen TS, Campbell JN et al (2008) Neuropathic pain: redefinition and a grading system for clinical and research purposes. Neurology 70(18):1630–1635

Causes of Endodontic Pain and Preventive Strategies

5

5.1 Causes of Endodontic Pain

Prior to discussing pain-preventive strategies, it is essential to understand basic pulp biology and the pulp's response to caries and other irritants.

Pulpal disease and concomitant pain is caused by caries, trauma, or as a result of restorative procedures. Although there are differences in the disease processes, ultimately microbiological factors are of critical importance.

Although caries is not the only cause of pulpal disease, understanding the principles of the pulp's dynamic response to caries is an important step in developing a pain-preventive strategy. Onset of pain subsequent to caries varies depending on a number of factors including presence of prior restorations, individual pain thresholds and host inflammatory and immune resistance. The response to advancing caries is so varied that even a carious exposure may occur without pain and is classified as asymptomatic irreversible pulpitis.

5.2 Caries

Even at early stages of the carious process, pulpal inflammation is seen in the pulp. Dentin permeability permits ingress of bacterial toxins into the pulp long before there is actual exposure of the pulp. This may or may not be accompanied by symptoms [29].

As caries progresses and the inflammatory process builds, the pulp's unique hard-tissue encasement has a role in ongoing tissue damage [29]. The repair of damaged pulp tissue is also affected by the limited capacity for drainage, and thin-walled vessels that are prone to collapse as intra-pulpal pressure builds. Intra-pulpal pressure increases as a consequence of inflammatory edema. As circulation shuts down, local areas of pulpal ischemia may expand quickly or over an extended period.

P.A. Rosenberg, *Endodontic Pain*,
DOI 10.1007/978-3-642-54701-0_5, © Springer-Verlag Berlin Heidelberg 2014

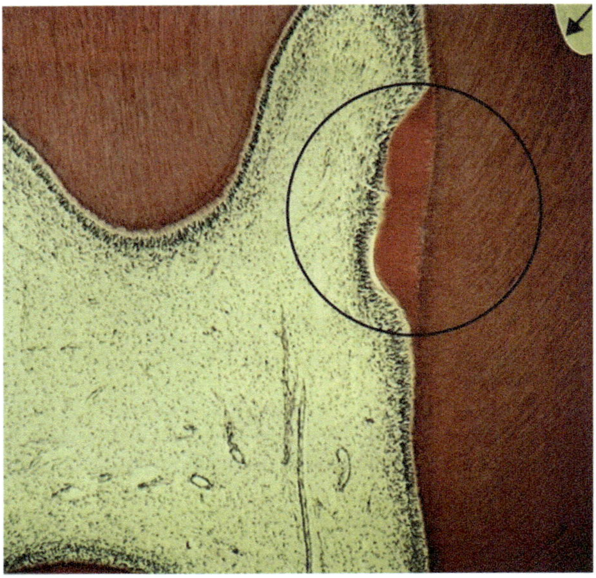

Fig. 5.1 Within the *circled area*, repair of dentin has occurred in response to a previous carious lesion. In the *upper right-hand corner*, the *arrow* indicates the result of a restoration

Radiographs provide little or no insight into the dynamics of the pulp's reaction to caries. However, a radiograph may reveal calcification of a chamber adjacent to a long-standing carious lesion. This reaction represents a defensive reaction of the pulp to an irritant that may ultimately complicate endodontic access. Similarly, long-term low-level inflammation may cause diffuse calcification in the root canal system that can impede endodontic instrumentation. Long-term inflammation can also sensitize nociceptors (pain receptors) and complicate local anesthesia (Fig. 5.1).

5.2.1 Host–Microbe Interactions in the Root Canal System

Multiple complex reactions involving attempts at repair and tissue breakdown may go on either asymptomatically or with pain ranging from mild to unbearable. Pulpitis, due to caries, has been described as an infection where the host reaction has the capacity to produce more damage than that caused simply by the effects of the microorganisms [29].

The outcome of the carious process, with or without pulp exposure, is subject to many variables. There are genetic factors involved in host response that are only now being elucidated. Age of the patient also plays a role in the capacity of tissue to respond to an insult. Prior dental experiences are also a factor. A tooth with periodontal disease and/or deep restorations often has a chronically inflamed pulp. Such a tooth is less likely to respond favorably to additional insults than a virgin tooth with healthy pulp and periodontal tissues. The clinician and his/her skills is also an important variable.

Pain, due to caries, is influenced by release of microbial metabolic products and growth factors from the dentin extracellular matrix. At the same time, the tubular characteristics of dentin and the extent of tubular sclerosis due to the reactionary response of the pulp-dentin complex affect the permeability of dentin. The degree of permeability affects the diffusion kinetics of the metabolic and degradation products into the pulp [31].

Response to Caries

There are vascular and cellular reactions as bacteria and toxins in the dentinal tubules approach the pulp. Increased vasodilation is caused by the release of vasoactive mediators including histamine. The initial cellular response of the pulp to carious exposure includes the infiltration of polymorphonuclear neutrophils (PMNs) and monocytes. Acute inflammation and tissue destruction follows, beginning with the formation of microabscesses and necrotic foci in the pulp, and eventually results in total pulp necrosis.

The process involves complex inflammatory and immune responses involving mediators and inflammatory cells. The periapical response to bacterial toxins and mediator release ultimately results in loss of bone and granuloma, periapical cyst, or abscess formation.

Pain is initiated by tissue damage that results in the release of chemical mediators. The mediators stimulate vasodilation and a cascade of reactions, which can result in formation of prostaglandins and other pain inducing mediators. Nonsteroidal anti-inflammatory medication (NSAIDs) can be used preemptively to block formation of pain inducing factors, such as prostaglandins. Please see Chap. 8 for a discussion of NSAIDs.

5.3 Low-Compliance System and Pain

The unique anatomy of the root canal system is an important complicating factor in patients' painful response to pulp damage. Elsewhere in the body (with the exception of the brain/cranium) as inflammation progresses fluid (edema) accumulates and causes swelling. "Unyielding walls of dentin" [48] is a descriptive phrase with a long history. It describes the fact that dentinal walls encasing the pulp do not allow for tissue expansion and prevents swelling. The relationship between the pulp and surrounding dentin walls has been characterized as a "low-compliance system." Due to the inability of the pulp to swell, inflammatory fluid accumulates in the confined space of the root canal, ultimately resulting in an increase of intra-pulpal pressure usually associated with pain.

Depending on its specific protein content, inflammatory fluid is termed a transudate, exudate, or pus. Pus is associated with an infectious process and contains variable amounts of dead polymorphonuclear leukocytes, bacterial elements, and blood.

Vasculature of the pulp is characterized by thin-walled vessels with rich collateralization and arterial–venous shunting [23]. As fluid accumulates in the canal system, and tissue pressure increases, areas of arterial vasculature collapse.

Ultimately venous drainage becomes overwhelmed and shuts down. Areas of the pulp deprived of circulation become ischemic and ultimately necrotic.

Clinical Tips

- The low-compliance system is a clinically meaningful concept. Endodontic pain is often associated with increased intra-pulpal or periapical tissue pressure.
- Emergency treatment: pulpotomy, extirpation of the pulp, and incision and drainage are all directed at reducing intra-pulpal and/or periapical tissue pressure as a means of eliminating pain.

5.3.1 Necrotic Pulp

Necrotic pulp is a dead tissue without functioning vasculature or structural integrity. It provides an ideal culture medium for bacterial colonization. In some cases this process unfolds rapidly and in others very slowly. Pain associated with the process is unpredictable and ranges from virtually intolerable to painless. Clinicians may see large carious exposures of long duration that have caused no pain in contrast to small carious pulp exposures that are extremely painful.

Histologically, it is common to find, within the same pulp, areas of acute inflammation, chronic inflammation, and necrosis. This is a dynamic process and the exposed pulp should be considered a tissue with numerous outcome possibilities. It may proceed to necrosis with or without symptoms or remain as an asymptomatic or symptomatic vital tissue for an indeterminate period of time. A better endodontic outcome is likely if pulp pathosis is treated before periapical pathosis develops.

Sensibility tests of a tooth with a carious exposure should be considered within the context of a dynamic tissue undergoing change. It is well established that pain and sensibility testing are not predictors of the histologic state of the pulp. Despite a vital response of a tooth to pulp testing, it should not necessarily be considered a normal pulp. Exposures and traumatized teeth with partial necrosis may have enough viable neural tissue remaining, to respond to provocation, and mislead a clinician. Ultimately, bacteria in the root canal system results in pulp necrosis.

5.3.2 A Classic Study

A classic study demonstrated the critical role of bacteria following a pulp exposure and the tissue's reaction to the presence of bacteria. Using a rat model, it was found that in the presence of bacteria, pulp tissue became partially necrotic within 8 days and completely necrotic with formation of periapical abscesses by 14 days. *This response was not seen in germ-free animals with pulpal exposures.*

At 32 days after pulp exposure in germ-free rats, an intact dentin bridge developed with normal pulp tissue beneath the newly formed dentin. Thus, bacterial infection of the pulp is the key etiologic factor for pulp necrosis. Endodontic therapy must include materials and methods that significantly reduce or eliminate bacteria [22].

This classic study is central to our understanding of endodontic success and failure.

Clinical procedures must be judged in the context of their ability to diminish or eliminate bacteria in the root canal system.

5.4 Trauma

Trauma causes a significant number of painful dental emergencies. Unlike the initial chronic inflammatory response to caries, the reaction to trauma may be immediate devitalization or may not become apparent for years. Excellent texts on the subject of trauma provide guidance for the clinician in treating patients with traumatic injuries. The reader may pursue in depth information on dental trauma in *Traumatic Dental Injuries* [2]. A useful website that links the best available evidence to treatment of traumatic injuries and expected outcomes can be accessed at www.dentaltraumaguide.org/.

Developed by Dr. Jens Ove Andreasen, the site is unique in its accessibility and value to all dentists treating traumatic injuries.

5.4.1 Restorative Factors

Restorative procedures can be the cause of pulpal problems. An important issue is microbial microleakage [41]. Penetration of microbes into the deeper sections of dentin and pulp can cause severe pain that may be difficult to diagnose. The durability of bonding and clinical success of adhesive restorations is an important area for continued research [9]. Iatrogenic factors during restorative procedures such as inadequate coolant and generation of heat are also potential causes of pulpal breakdown.

It is common to have a patient complain of thermal sensitivity following a restorative procedure. A key question for the clinician involves determination of whether or not pulpitis and resulting thermal sensitivity is reversible or irreversible. The patient's level of pain and its duration are subjective findings but are important factors in judging the probability of reversibility or irreversibility of the process.

Clinical Tips

- Sensitivity to percussion, if hyper-occlusion can be ruled out, is a critical sign indicating that pulpal inflammation has extended from the pulp into the periodontal ligament. This biological event usually signals an irreversible pulpitis.

The aim of the wise is not to secure pleasure but to avoid pain Socrates

5.5 Pain-Preventive Strategies

5.5.1 Preoperative Strategy

Biologically based preoperative, intraoperative, and postoperative strategies can have a preventive effect on patient's pain and endodontic experience. A pain-preventive or preemptive strategy is a multifaceted plan directed at prevention *or* reduction of intraoperative and postoperative pain. The strategy includes anxiety reduction, profound local anesthesia, biologically based operative and postoperative procedures, and preemptive use of analgesics.

Clinical Tips

- Pain is more difficult to eliminate after it has been established.
- A pain-preventive strategy is based on a preemptive approach using appropriate local anesthetics (longer lasting), preemptive analgesia, anxiety reduction techniques, and clinical strategies.

5.5.2 Pain: Predisposing Factors

Most clinicians have treated two patients of the same gender with similar teeth and medical/dental histories. The teeth are treated using the same clinical approach but one patient has a smooth postoperative course while another experiences complications including severe pain and swelling. The clinician often looks for an iatrogenic cause of the pain. While iatrogenic factors often exist, there is increasing evidence that there are other factors that may predispose some patients to complications.

This section will examine the potential role of predisposing factors and comorbidities including genetics, gender, and anxiety.

5.5.3 Comorbidities

A comorbidity has been defined as a concomitant but unrelated pathologic or disease process [1].

For example, it has been suggested that patients with chronic pain conditions, elsewhere in the body, may be predisposed to prolonged pain after apparently successful endodontic therapy [40]. Patients with a high level of anxiety or chronic facial pain problems are examples of comorbidities that may affect the patient's experience during and after endodontic therapy. A patient's sex may also be a factor as there is evidence that females may be predisposed to certain painful conditions.

5.5.4 Predictors of Endodontic Pain

Although endodontic treatment can be virtually pain free during the procedure itself, some patients may experience varying degrees of pain following treatment.

It is helpful for the clinician to recognize factors that are predictive of postoperative pain. That information may influence the endodontic treatment plan. For example, a decision concerning single or multi-visit treatment could be influenced by knowledge of predisposing factors [20].

Studies have investigated postoperative endodontic pain and reported an incidence of moderate to severe pain in the range of 15–25 % [10, 21, 37]. A prospective clinical study reported that 57 % of patients reported no pain after debridement and shaping of the root canal system, although 21 % had slight pain, 15 % had moderate pain, and 7 % had severe pain [17].

Although some patients may experience moderate to severe pain after endodontic treatment, few experience what is now commonly referred to as a flare-up or a postoperative problem requiring an unscheduled visit with unplanned treatment intervention to manage the patient's symptoms [50]. Patients with a flare-up usually describe severe pain, swelling, or the sensation of pressure in their mandible or maxilla within 1 or 2 days of treatment.

The incidence of flare-up varies across studies and ranges from about 2 to 20 % of patients, with the higher prevalence generally reported in older studies using classic cleaning and shaping techniques [5, 46, 47]. Differences in experimental design prevent direct comparison of those research results, but the presence of preoperative pain or mechanical allodynia (reduced mechanical pain threshold or percussion sensitivity) was a positive predictor of postoperative pain in more than 15 studies involving more than 6,600 patients.

Other factors were more variable in their predictive value of postoperative pain. In a retrospective study, the dental records of 1,000 patients who had nonsurgical root canal treatment and experienced no flare-ups (i.e., unscheduled return visits) were compared with the records of 1,000 patients who experienced flare-ups after the cleansing and shaping of their necrotic root canals [45]. The results showed that factors such as presence of preoperative pain, tooth type, sex, age, history of allergy, and retreatment were significantly predictive for the incidence of flare-up, although intra-canal medicaments, systemic disease, and establishment of patency of the apical foramen had no significant relation to the incidence of flare-ups. Specifically, the highest incidence of flare-ups was associated with mandibular teeth, retreatment procedures, females over the age of 40, and patients with a history of allergies [45].

5.6 The Influence of Other Factors on Patients Pain: Genetics, Sex, and Anxiety

Based on the best available evidence, it seems likely that there are factors that predispose a patient to pain. These factors may alter the patient's pain threshold as well as their response to tissue injury and treatment. Some of the factors are apparent such as the patient's sex, while others like the patient's genetic background remain unknown to clinicians. This is likely to change in the future (Figs. 5.2 and 5.3).

The subject of predisposing factors is undergoing scrutiny, and it is reasonable to assume that there will be further elucidation of important predictors of pain. It is interesting to consider the future and the implications of increasing knowledge in the area of genetics and the role the patient's sex may have on our prevention and treatment of pain.

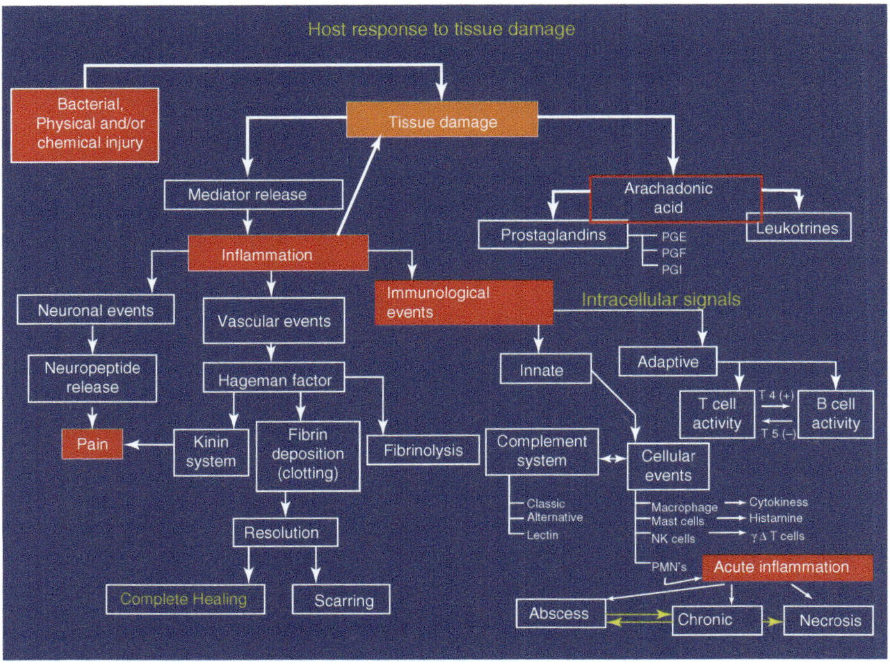

Fig. 5.2 Dynamic response of a patient to tissue damage

Fig. 5.3 Comorbidities can be complicating factors during endodontic treatment

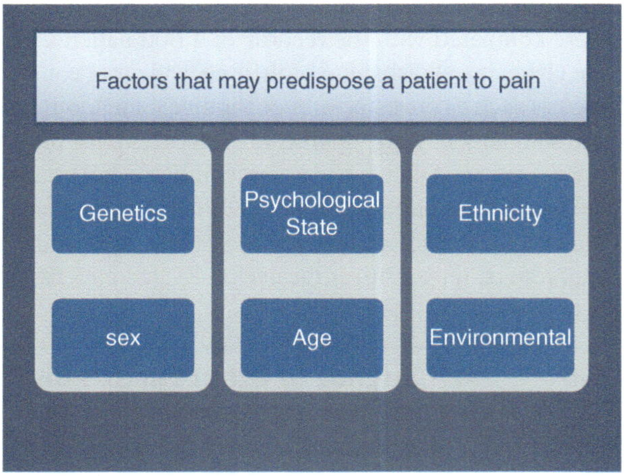

5.6.1 Genetics

The role of genetics is an entirely new variable for dentists to consider. Genetics may play a role in predisposing some patients to a variety of complications including pain, poor healing, and abscess formation. Genetic factors may also be important in determining how a person responds to specific drugs. Considering the role of genetics in endodontics is highly complex and at an early stage of development.

Increasingly, current endodontic literature provides examples of how genetics may influence endodontic symptoms and outcomes. Findings suggest that specific markers associated with the pro-inflammatory regulator Il-1B, a key regulator of host response, may contribute to increased susceptibility to periapical pathosis [32]. It has also been suggested that genetic factors are associated with a susceptibility to develop symptomatic dental abscesses [11].

Numerous genes are involved with the pharmacokinetics and dynamics of opioids thus complicating the issue of genetics and patient's response to an opioid. A variety of genetic polymorphisms clearly influence pain perception and behavior in response to pain. The response to analgesics differs depending on complex factors including the pain modality and the potential for repeated noxious stimuli, the opioid prescribed, and even its route of administration [49].

The Human Genome Project has contributed to the possibility of the development of drugs specific for individualized therapy. It seems clear that genetic variations influence both the efficacy and side effects of drugs used to treat pain. A study examined genetic and environmental contributions to variability in pain sensitivity and responsiveness to opioid analgesics. Findings indicated that inter-individual variance in responsiveness to opioids is at least in part due to genetics [3]. More than 20 genes affecting pain sensitivity in humans or interindividual variability have been identified. While at this time some of the data is conflicting, it is exciting to think about what the future of genetics may mean to endodontists of the future [33].

For example, it has been suggested that markers in MMP3 and MMP2 genes could predict host susceptibility to developing periapical lesions and the healing response. Genetic predisposition in specific genes can contribute to persistent apical periodontitis [30]. It seems likely that an understanding of the genetic basis of endodontic pain perception will advance our pharmacologic management of postoperative pain.

These preliminary findings point to a rich complex of factors associated with patient's pain and treatment outcomes. It is possible that as more information is collected, we will be better able to identify those patients predisposed to pain and have a diminished capacity for healing.

5.6.2 Sex and Gender

Terminology

Although biological sex exerts a major influence on a person's gender identity, "sex" and "gender" are not interchangeable terms. The term "sex" refers to biologically based differences, while the term "gender" refers to socially based phenomena. If research subjects are to be categorized by anatomic features (chromosomes, reproductive organs), it is appropriate to describe the study as one of "sex differences."

In contrast, if additional measures of masculinity/femininity or gender identity are used to describe subjects, then the term "gender differences" is appropriate [19].

Pain Responses: Men and Women

During the last 10–15 years, there is a growing body of evidence indicating that there are substantial sex differences in clinical and experimental pain responses for women and men [15]. It seems that women are at a substantially greater risk for many clinical pain conditions. An extensive review reported that a survey of the currently available epidemiological and laboratory data indicates that there is overwhelming evidence for clinical and experimental sex differences in pain. Numerous reasons for these findings have been given, including hormonal and genetically driven sex differences in brain neurochemistry [49]. Furthermore, some highly prevalent chronic pain syndromes that are found in both sexes (including chronic fatigue syndrome, fibromyalgia, interstitial cystitis, and temporomandibular disorder) occur overwhelmingly more often (in more than 80 % of cases in which treatment is sought) in women.

Interestingly, it was observed that natural redheaded women required 19 % more desflurane (volatile anesthetic) than women with dark hair. Initially this observation was reported anecdotally, but the observation was investigated and it was determined that red hair in women was the result of a genetic variant and also a distinct phenotype associated with anesthetic requirements in humans [26]. In 2005, it was found that there was increased thermal sensitivity and reduced subcutaneous lidocaine efficacy in redheads. However, another study was unable to replicate those findings when inferior alveolar nerve blocks were evaluated [12].

5.7 Recent Research: Probability of Pain

A clinical study investigated the probability of the incidence, intensity, duration, and triggering of post-endodontic pain, considering factors related to the patient (age, gender, medical evaluation) and the affected tooth (location, number of canals, pulp vitality, preoperative pain, periapical radiolucencies, previous emergency access, and presence of occlusal contacts) [4].

Independent factors were recorded during the treatment, and characteristics of post-endodontic pain (incidence, intensity, type, and duration) were surveyed through questionnaires. Of the 500 questionnaires, 374 were properly returned and split in two groups for two different statistical purposes: 316 cases were used to adjust the logistic regression models to predict each characteristic of post-endodontic pain using predictive factors, and the remaining 58 cases were used to test the validity of each model [4].

The predictive models determined that:

- The incidence of *post-endodontic pain was significantly lower* when the treated tooth was not a molar ($p = 0.003$).
- Demonstrated periapical radiolucencies ($p = 0.003$).

- Had no history of previous pain ($p=0.006$) or emergency endodontic treatment ($p=0.045$).
- Had no occlusal contact ($p<0.0001$).

The probability of experiencing moderate or severe pain was higher with increasing age ($p=0.09$) and in mandibular teeth ($p=0.045$). The probability of pain lasting more than 2 days was increased with age ($p=0.1$) and decreased in males ($p=0.007$) and when a radiolucent lesion was present on radiographs ($p=0.1$) [4].

5.7.1 Incidence

- The research results found that the *most influential factor* in *predicting post-endodontic pain is the absence of occlusal contacts*, with an odds ratio = 3.3 (95 % Confidence Interval = 1.9–5.6). This odds ratio is 1.6 times higher than the next factor in order of importance (presence of preoperative pain).
- It was predicted that the patient with the highest probability of developing post-endodontic pain had previously experienced pain in a molar with prior endodontic treatment, no apical radiolucency, and occlusal contacts.
- In contrast, a hypothetical patient with no previous pain in an incisor, a cuspid, or a bicuspid with an apical radiolucency and free from occlusion will have a 0.07 probability of developing post-endodontic pain. Those odds would be a very good bet [4].

5.7.2 Research Bias

A recent review, determined that at least 79 % of animal studies published in the journal *Pain* over the preceding 10 years included male subjects only, with 8 % of studies on females only, and another 4 % explicitly designed to test for sex differences (the rest did not specify). There is a substantially greater prevalence of many clinical pain conditions in women vs. men and growing evidence for sex differences in sensitivity to experimental pain and to analgesics. It is invalid to assume that data obtained in male subjects will generalize to females. In both preclinical and clinical studies, a comparison of both sexes would further our understanding of individual differences in sensitivity to pain and analgesia, thus improving our ability to treat and prevent pain in all people [19].

Determining whether women have different sensitivity to pain or analgesia compared with men is complicated by the hormonal cyclicity of women. In most clinical research studies, men have been used as subjects and women have been largely excluded. The reason for this selectivity is based on the complexity of women's menstrual cycle and the effect (both pro- and anti-inflammatory) of estrogen. At least 79 % of animal studies published in the journal *Pain* during a recent 10-year period included males only [19].

The significance of this research bias cannot be overestimated. It is becoming increasingly clear that one cannot always draw conclusions from male-dominated research and apply them to women.

5.7.3 Anxiety

The level of anxiety varies among patients, but to some degree, all are fearful about root canal therapy and pain. The media, negative previous dental experiences, and warnings from other patients add to the patient's anxiety. There are over 200 studies indicating that preemptive behavioral intervention to decrease anxiety before and after surgery reduces postoperative pain intensity and intake of analgesics and accelerates recovery [7].

5.7.4 Clinical Research

- An implant study examined the relationship between anxiety and acute pain perception of patients experienced at different stages of the procedure.
- It was determined that pain experienced by patients was best predicted by their *anxiety* at each time point.
- Patient's anxiety was significantly associated with the subject's *expectation of experiencing pain* during the procedure [13].
- It is likely that those findings could be extended to endodontics.

Clinical Tips

- The previous research findings point to the importance of spending a few moments, prior to treatment, explaining your pain-preventive strategy that includes waiting sufficient time for profound anesthesia, supplementary injections, and use of preemptive pain medication.

5.8 Avoiding Treatment

Avoidance of dental treatment due to anxiety has been associated with significant deterioration of oral and dental health. Even at the diagnostic stage, severe anxiety may confuse the process. Several studies support the hypothesis that pain or fear of pain is a primary source of anxiety as well as an obstacle to seeking dental care [6, 25, 53]. Also, highly anxious patients appear to be more sensitive to pain [24]. High levels of anxiety have been found to negatively affect clinical procedures including local anesthesia [34].

It has been demonstrated that dental anxiety and expectation of pain had a profound effect on patient's ability to understand information provided [14]. A study found that 40 % of patients who had minor oral surgery did not remember receiving both written and verbal instructions, contributing to 67 % noncompliance with antibiotic prescriptions.

5.8.1 Behavioral Modification

There are important steps to take even *before* local anesthesia is administered. In a landmark medical study it was found that pretreatment discussion of surgical treatments and associated discomfort reduced by 50 % the need for posttreatment morphine and reduced the time to discharge [7]. More than 200 studies indicate that preemptive behavioral intervention decreases anxiety before and after surgery, reduces posttreatment pain intensity and intake of analgesics, and accelerates recovery [7].

A calm setting, reassurance by the clinician and explanation of the treatment plan, as well as a discussion about pain-preventive strategies are important before treatment starts [35]. Written as well as a verbal description of the proposed treatment are helpful. It may also be of value to have a family member or friend accompany the patient for a discussion of the treatment plan.

Discussing the patient's past dental experiences provides insight into the level of the patient's anxiety. All dentists have heard the following, "I have had root canal therapy done before, and it was the worst day of my life." The statement, or others like it, is important. It provides insight into the patient's emotional status before starting treatment. At the same time it represents an opportunity for a dentist to discuss his/her approach to treatment and to develop a new trusting patient.

There is research that links anxiety to inadequate local anesthesia and the level of pain experienced by a patient [36]. A link seems to exist between a patient's level of anxiety and how they react to an endodontic procedure. As the level of anxiety increases the patient's pain threshold drops. This negative cycle must be recognized and addressed.

Some clinicians take a pharmacologic approach to patient's anxiety. However, the vast majority of patients can be managed by using a sensitive, caring approach to a patient's fears and concerns. A patient/dentist conversation can be powerful medicine in most cases. The dialogue should include a description of profound anesthesia and reassurance that the clinician uses an array of pain-preventive strategies that did not exist years ago.

Most patients experience a meaningful reduction in their level of anxiety after a supportive preoperative conversation with their dentist about the procedure. They should be given an opportunity to express their fears and the clinician should provide information about his/her pain-preventive strategy. The discussion should include information about the depth of local anesthesia to be achieved, preemptive use of analgesics, postoperative medication, and availability of the practitioner to the patient after-hours. The strength of the clinician–patient relationship is important when providing effective treatment for pain. Pain treatment is never about the intervention alone, but about the clinician and patient working together [39].

It is likely that the vast majority of patients can be helped to overcome their anxiety by the use a positive preoperative interaction with the dentist and staff. This confidence building will pay dividends during treatment and in the postoperative period. It will also help with patient compliance and the use of analgesics and antibiotics.

5.9 Older Patients

Older patients are a growing segment of the population [28]. It is estimated that by 2020, one in six Americans will be 65 years of age or older. Compared with younger patients, older patients tend to have more medical problems and take more medications. One half of those older than 65 years of age have two or more chronic illnesses, and the elderly take one third of all prescription medications.

Of persons aged 65 or older, only 39 % report that their health is either good or excellent. Older patients often suffer from multiple comorbid conditions of variable degree, with an increased frequency of nonspecific signs or symptoms, drug interactions, or side effects. Frailty, cognitive impairment, and physical disabilities are common in aged patients. It is important to be sensitive to these realities and to approach diagnosis, treatment planning, and treatment in the older patient with extra consideration and caution [28].

5.10 Adjunctive Pharmacotherapy

Adjunctive pharmacotherapy (anxiolytic drugs) is useful in the management of some patient's with moderate to severe anxiety during endodontic treatment. Anxiety reduction can reduce the response to potentially painful stimuli during treatment and decrease the tendency of the patient to recall the endodontic procedure as unpleasant [16].

Clinical Tips

Strategies to Reduce Anxiety

- Establishment of good rapport and trust is of importance.
- Allow the patient to ask questions and encourage frank and open discussion concerning the procedure.
- Explaining what is to be done before treatment is initiated often helps put the patient at ease.

- Short morning appointments may be better tolerated than appointments may be better tolerated than appointments later in the day.
- In patients with pronounced anxiety or fear about a planned dental procedure, oral premedication with an anxiolytic or sedative drug 1 h before an appointment can be useful. In addition, an anxiolytic or sedative can be prescribed the night before the appointment to ensure a good night's rest.
- A commonly used agent for this purpose is triazolam (Halcion, Pfizer), a short-acting benzodiazepine. Other drugs such as diazepam, oxazepam, lorazepam, or hydroxyzine also may be used. If an anxiolytic or sedative is prescribed, patients should be cautioned not to drive or operate machinery while under the influence of the drug. Intraoperative monitoring by pulse oximetry is recommended for those who are sedated with oral medication.
- Injection of local anesthetic is the procedure that most patients fear; therefore, every effort should be made to avoid pain during administration.
- It is important to keep the needle and syringe out of the patient's sight.
- Topical anesthetic should be applied, followed by slow advancement of the needle and slow injection of the solution after aspiration. Adequate time should then be allowed after injection to ensure adequate anesthesia before the start of work.
- The best means of determining the existence of profound anesthesia is to provoke the tooth using the chief complaint as a test. Thus the patient with a chief complaint of sensitivity to percussion should have the tooth percussed. Absence of pain indicates profound anesthesia. Pain would indicate that additional steps must be taken to achieve profound anesthesia. These steps are described in Chap. 6.

5.10.1 Nitrous Oxide

Mild to moderate anxiety can usually be managed with the use of nitrous oxide [43]. Some clinicians find the mask to be cumbersome, but the benefits of nitrous oxide outweigh the inconvenience of the apparatus. When radiographs are required the mask can be removed briefly to facilitate the procedure. Some highly anxious patients may require more than nitrous oxide [8] (Fig. 5.4).

5.10.2 Anxiety and Conscious Sedation

Triazolam (Halcion, Pfizer) has been shown to reduce anxiety, and some believe that it may secondarily increase the success rate of the inferior alveolar nerve block (IANB) [27]. However, a prospective, randomized, double-blind, placebo-controlled study evaluated the effect of sublingual triazolam on the efficacy of the IANB in

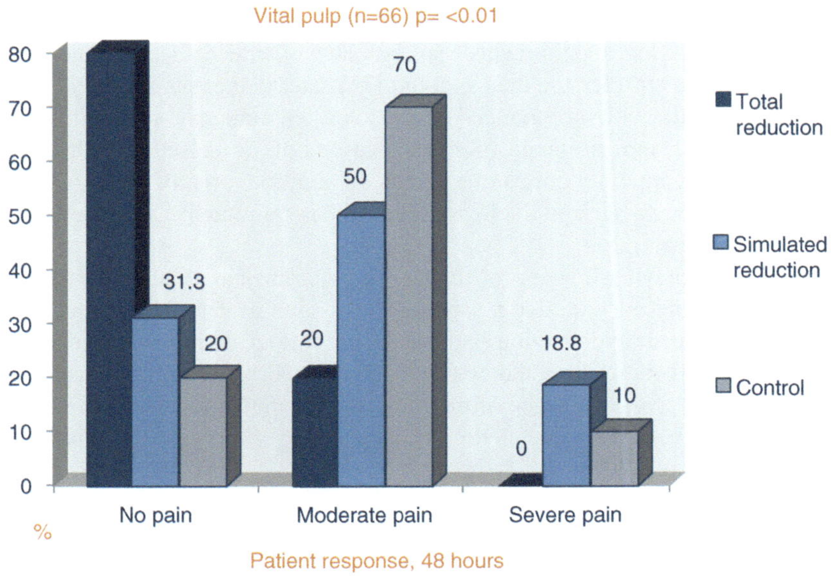

Fig. 5.4 Result of occlusal reduction in teeth with vital pulps undergoing endodontic treatment following cleaning/shaping

patients with irreversible pulpitis. A sublingual triazolam dose of 0.25 mg did not increase the success of the IANB in patients with irreversible pulpitis.

Even when using conscious sedation, profound local anesthesia is still required to eliminate pain during dental treatment [52]. Pain in sedated, unconscious patients is underreported and undertreated [38]. It was demonstrated that sedated, unconscious patients detect, experience, and respond to pain but are unable to remember the painful event due to their unconscious state.

5.11 Local Anesthesia

Local anesthesia, discussed in Chap. 6, must be mentioned here as part of a basic pain-preventive strategy. The injection of local anesthetic represents a fearsome moment for most patients. It is an especially important moment for the patient because it represents the initial operative experience following the dentist–patient dialogue concerning dentist's focus on pain prevention. It is discouraging for a patient to experience a painful injection following reassurance from the dentist about his/her gentleness. Starting treatment without adequate anesthesia is a predictor of intraoperative and postoperative pain and an unhappy patient.

5.11.1 Injection Pain

An injection is highly technique sensitive and is influenced by a number of human and mechanical factors.

A dental injection may be the most universally feared procedure. Some of the fear is based on past experience, hearsay, and experience with injections elsewhere in the body. Many patients base a significant part of their assessment of the dentist on how gentle they are during this procedure. There are important points to review associated with injections that can be helpful to the clinician seeking to determine what evidence exists concerning what techniques are or are not meaningful in pain reduction.

An excellent textbook on successful local anesthesia is available. It describes research and clinical information of value to clinicians [36].

Clinical Tips

- A numb lip is not good evidence of profound local anesthesia.
- Profound anesthesia takes time.
- The best test of profound anesthesia is to repeat the provoking stimulus that initially caused pain.
- Thus if the chief complaint was cold sensitivity, the clinician should apply a cold stimulus to the tooth. If pain persists, supplementary injections may be required.

5.11.2 Occlusal Reduction as a Pain-Preventive Strategy

Following endodontic instrumentation, when specific indicators are present, an important evidence-based pain-preventive strategy is occlusal reduction. However, there may be restorative considerations, such as a new crown or fixed prosthesis that may prevent implementation of that strategy.

Occlusal reduction has been found to be highly effective in cases that are vital, sensitive to percussion, have a history of pain, and are without a periapical lesion. An extensive clinical study validated that there were specific clinical indicators for occlusal reduction and found it to be statistically significant as a pain-preventive strategy in appropriate cases [42] (Figs. 5.5 and 5.6).

Clinical Tips

- In appropriate cases occlusal reduction is a significant pain-preventive strategy.
- Patients with vital teeth, preoperative pain, without periapical lesions, and sensitivity to percussion are candidates for occlusal reduction unless there are restorative considerations that intervene.
- Occlusal reduction means the relief of centric occlusion and all excursions.
- At emergency visits, following initial endodontic treatment, most patients, especially those with a history of preoperative pain and/or percussion sensitivity, respond well to occlusal reduction and experience a dramatic reduction in pain.
- Leaving such teeth in occlusion often results in continuation of pain following endodontic instrumentation.

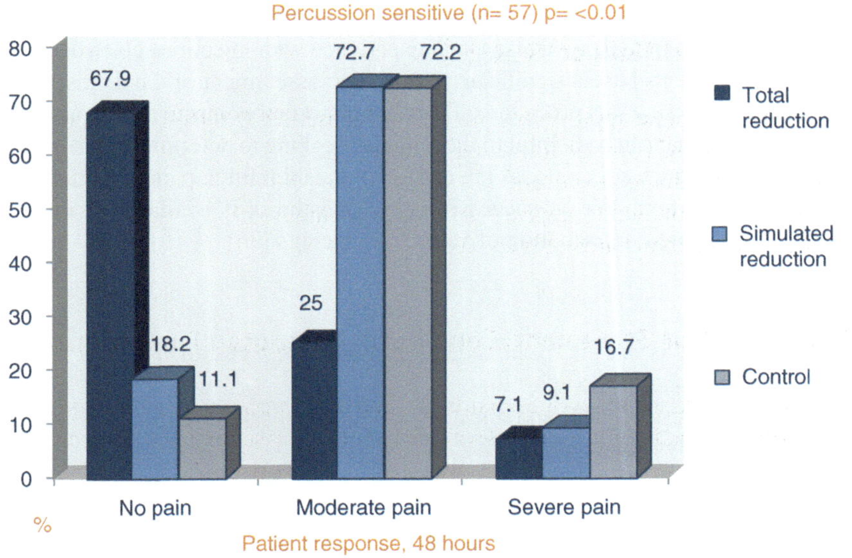

Fig. 5.5 Response of percussion sensitive teeth to occlusal reduction following cleaning/shaping

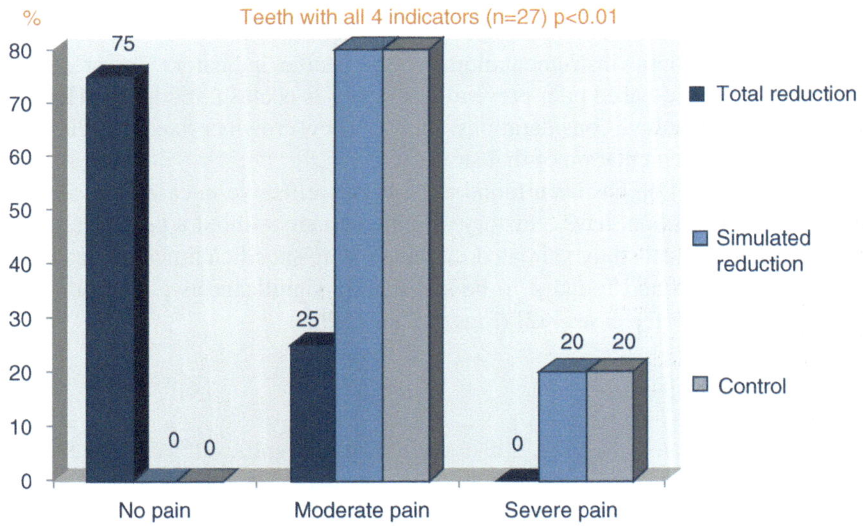

Fig. 5.6 Response of vital teeth, percussion sensitive, history of pain, and no radiolucency to occlusal reduction

Additional Recent Occlusal/Pain Research

A recent prospective clinical study investigated predictive models of pain following root canal treatment determined that "the most influential factor in predicting the incidence of post-endodontic pain is the absence of occlusal contacts" ($P<0.0001$) [4].

This research further validates the importance of occlusal reduction in cases that meet the appropriate criteria.

5.11.3 Preoperative Pain: Influence on Tooth Survival

It was found that the influence of preoperative pain on tooth survival changed over time as its effect declined at around 22 months following treatment. This finding may be explained by the fact that preoperative pain is a predictor for postoperative [51] and chronic persistent [40] pain following root canal treatment.

In some instances, the preoperative pain may be of non-endodontic origin and therefore persists after root canal treatment [40]. Accurate diagnosis of an odontogenic or non-odontogenic cause of pain is critical in the patient's follow-up care. A diagnostic error may cause patients to seek additional unnecessary endodontic treatment or tooth extraction.

In some cases, preoperative pain of endodontic origin may persist following treatment, as a result of peripheral or central sensitization. Therefore, effective pain diagnosis and management of patients presenting with preoperative pain or medical conditions is crucial.

Intra-visit Pain

Intra-visit pain, ranging from mild to severe, can occur in both vital (irreversible pulpitis) and non-vital (necrotic) cases. In vital cases, the most common cause of intra-visit pain is inaccurate measurement control and/or failure to maintain an accurate measurement during cleaning and shaping. Instrumenting significantly short of the measurement or beyond that point is a predictor of intra-visit pain.

In non-vital cases pain/swelling usually results from pushing microbial debris from the canal into the periapical tissues. The result is an acute inflammatory and immune response altering the host–parasite balance.

Depending on the specifics of each case, appropriate clinical and analgesic/antibiotic strategy should be provided. The treatment selected is dependent on the clinician's understanding of the cause of the problem.

Please see Chap. 7 for a discussion of flare-ups and Chap. 8 for a review of analgesics and antibiotics.

Post-obturation Pain

Reports of the incidence of post-obturation pain vary; however, most show that the pain tends to occur in the first 24 h [21, 44]. There is a correlation between the level of obturation and pain incidence, with overextension associated with the highest incidence of discomfort [18, 21].

Post-obturation pain is also related to pre-obturation pain. Levels of pain reported after obturation tend to correlate with levels of pain before the appointment [21, 44]. If basic precautions are followed, there is usually not a need for an emergency visit following obturation. However, mild to moderate pain after obturation is common and can most often be treated successfully with analgesics for 24–48 h.

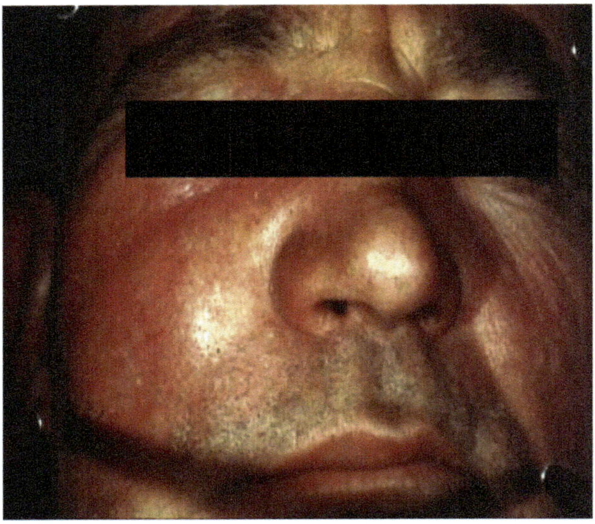

Fig. 5.7 Cellulitis extending into the buccinator and infraorbital spaces. A severe response of this type signals the need for removal of the root canal filling, antibiotic therapy, and retreatment. Depending on the nature of intraoral swelling, incision and drainage may also be indicated

Clinical Tips

- Postponing obturation until the tooth is comfortable is the best means of preventing postoperative complications.
- Patients should be advised that mild post-obturation pain may occur and can usually be easily treated. Preemptive use of analgesics can be helpful in the days following obturation.
- Reassurance concerning the availability of emergency care is helpful in allaying patient's fears.

5.11.4 More Serious Complications Following Obturation

Some patients develop more serious post-obturation complications characterized by severe pain and/or swelling. These patients must be seen for evaluation and treatment. A basic question for the clinician involves whether or not to remove the root canal filling (Fig. 5.7).

In most cases, if the filling is assessed to be acceptable, it does not have to be removed. However, in the presence of significant swelling, especially if it is increasing and or the patient has fever, removal of the filling may enable the clinician to establish drainage through the tooth.

Removal of the filling and retreatment and perhaps apical surgery is always indicated when prior treatment has been inadequate. In cases that exacerbate sometime after endodontic therapy has been completed, retreatment decisions may be complicated by presence of a post or other restorative concerns.

If the root canal treatment is acceptable, incision and drainage of a significant fluctuant swelling can be helpful. Diffuse mild swelling or "puffiness" usually resolves without further treatment. The use of antibiotics, in appropriate cases (see Chap. 8) may be seen as an adjunct and not curative in cases that require removal of the filling and retreatment.

References

1. Editors of the American Heritage Dictionary (2007) The American Heritage Medical Dictionary. Houghton Mifflin Company, Boston
2. Andreasen JO (2011) Traumatic dental injuries: a manual. Wiley-Blackwell, West Sussex
3. Angst MS, Phillips NG, Drover DR et al (2012) Pain sensitivity and opioid analgesia: a pharmacogenomic twin study. Pain 153(7):1397–1409
4. Arias A, De La Macorra JC, Hidalgo JJ et al (2013) Predictive models of pain following root canal treatment: a prospective clinical study. Int Endod J 46(8):784–793
5. Barnett F, Tronstad L (1989) The incidence of flare-ups following endodontic treatment. J Dent Res 68:1253
6. Binkley CJ, Beacham A, Neace W et al (2009) Genetic variations associated with red hair color and fear of dental pain, anxiety regarding dental care and avoidance of dental care. J Am Dent Assoc 140(7):896–905
7. Carr DB, Goudas LC (1999) Acute pain. Lancet 353(9169):2051–2058
8. Carter LE, McNeil DW, Vowles KE et al (2002) Effects of emotion on pain reports, tolerance and physiology. Pain Res Manag 7(1):21–30
9. Carvalho RM, Manso AP, Geraldeli S et al (2012) Durability of bonds and clinical success of adhesive restorations. Dent Mater 28(1):72–86
10. Clem WH (1970) Posttreatment endodontic pain. J Am Dent Assoc 81(5):1166–1170
11. De Sa AR, Moreira PR, Xavier GM et al (2007) Association of CD14, IL1B, IL6, IL10 and TNFA functional gene polymorphisms with symptomatic dental abscesses. Int Endod J 40(7):563–572
12. Droll B, Drum M, Nusstein J et al (2012) Anesthetic efficacy of the inferior alveolar nerve block in red-haired women. J Endod 38(12):1564–1569
13. Eli I, Schwartz-Arad D, Baht R et al (2003) Effect of anxiety on the experience of pain in implant insertion. Clin Oral Implants Res 14(1):115–118
14. Eli I, Schwartz-Arad D, Bartal Y (2008) Anxiety and ability to recognize clinical information in dentistry. J Dent Res 87(1):65–68
15. Fillingim RB, King CD, Ribeiro-Dasilva MC et al (2009) Sex, gender, and pain: a review of recent clinical and experimental findings. J Pain 10(5):447–485
16. Gedney JJ, Logan H, Baron RS (2003) Predictors of short-term and long-term memory of sensory and affective dimensions of pain. J Pain 4(2):47–55
17. Georgopoulou M, Anastassiadis P, Sykaras S (1986) Pain after chemomechanical preparation. Int Endod J 19(6):309–314
18. Gesi A, Hakeberg M, Warfvinge J et al (2006) Incidence of periapical lesions and clinical symptoms after pulpectomy–a clinical and radiographic evaluation of 1- versus 2-session treatment. Oral Surg Oral Med Oral Pathol Oral Radiol Endod 101(3):379–388
19. Greenspan JD, Craft RM, Leresche L et al (2007) Studying sex and gender differences in pain and analgesia: a consensus report. Pain 132(Suppl 1):S26–S45
20. Hargreaves KM, Cohen S, Berman LH (2011) Cohen's pathways of the pulp. Mosby Elsevier, St. Louis
21. Harrison JW, Baumgartner JC, Svec TA (1983) Incidence of pain associated with clinical factors during and after root canal therapy. Part 2. Postobturation pain. J Endod 9(10):434–438
22. Kakehashi S, Stanley HR, Fitzgerald RJ (1965) The effects of surgical exposures of dental pulps in germ-free and conventional laboratory rats. Oral Surg Oral Med Oral Pathol 20: 340–349

23. Kim S (1985) Microcirculation of the dental pulp in health and disease. J Endod 11(11): 465–471
24. Klages U, Kianifard S, Ulusoy O et al (2006) Anxiety sensitivity as predictor of pain in patients undergoing restorative dental procedures. Community Dent Oral Epidemiol 34(2):139–145
25. Lahmann C, Schoen R, Henningsen P et al (2008) Brief relaxation versus music distraction in the treatment of dental anxiety: a randomized controlled clinical trial. J Am Dent Assoc 139(3):317–324
26. Liem EB, Lin CM, Suleman MI et al (2004) Anesthetic requirement is increased in redheads. Anesthesiology 101(2):279–283
27. Lindemann M, Reader A, Nusstein J et al (2008) Effect of sublingual triazolam on the success of inferior alveolar nerve block in patients with irreversible pulpitis. J Endod 34(10): 1167–1170
28. Little JW, Falace DA, Miller C et al (2012) Dental management of the medically compromised patient. Mosby, St. Louis
29. Martin FE (2003) Carious pulpitis: microbiological and histopathological considerations. Aust Endod J 29(3):134–137
30. Menezes-Silva R, Khaliq S, Deeley K et al (2012) Genetic susceptibility to periapical disease: conditional contribution of MMP2 and MMP3 genes to the development of periapical lesions and healing response. J Endod 38(5):604–607
31. Mjor IA (2009) Dentin permeability: the basis for understanding pulp reactions and adhesive technology. Braz Dent J 20(1):3–16
32. Morsani JM, Aminoshariae A, Han YW et al (2011) Genetic predisposition to persistent apical periodontitis. J Endod 37(4):455–459
33. Muralidharan A, Smith MT (2011) Pain, analgesia and genetics. J Pharm Pharmacol 63(11):1387–1400
34. Nakai Y, Milgrom P, Mancl L et al (2000) Effectiveness of local anesthesia in pediatric dental practice. J Am Dent Assoc 131(12):1699–1705
35. Ng SK, Chau AW, Leung WK (2004) The effect of pre-operative information in relieving anxiety in oral surgery patients. Community Dent Oral Epidemiol 32(3):227–235
36. Nusstein JM, Reader A, Drum M (2010) Local anesthesia strategies for the patient with a "hot" tooth. Dent Clin North Am 54(2):237–247
37. O'keefe EM (1976) Pain in endodontic therapy: preliminary study. J Endod 2(10):315–319
38. Payen JF, Bru O, Bosson JL et al (2001) Assessing pain in critically ill sedated patients by using a behavioral pain scale. Crit Care Med 29(12):2258–2263
39. Pizzo PA, Clark NM (2012) Alleviating suffering 101–pain relief in the United States. N Engl J Med 366(3):197–199
40. Polycarpou N, Ng YL, Canavan D et al (2005) Prevalence of persistent pain after endodontic treatment and factors affecting its occurrence in cases with complete radiographic healing. Int Endod J 38(3):169–178
41. Roberts HW, Pashley DH (2012) Hydrostatic pulpal pressure effect upon microleakage. Am J Dent 25(1):49–53
42. Rosenberg PA, Babick PJ, Schertzer L et al (1998) The effect of occlusal reduction on pain after endodontic instrumentation. J Endod 24(7):492–496
43. Saxen MA, Newton CW (1999) Managing the endodontic patient with disabling anxiety or phobia. J Indiana Dent Assoc 78(4):21–23
44. Torabinejad M, Dorn SO, Eleazer PD et al (1994) Effectiveness of various medications on postoperative pain following root canal obturation. J Endod 20(9):427–431
45. Torabinejad M, Kettering JD, McGraw JC et al (1988) Factors associated with endodontic interappointment emergencies of teeth with necrotic pulps. J Endod 14(5):261–266
46. Trope M (1990) Relationship of intracanal medicaments to endodontic flare-ups. Endod Dent Traumatol 6(5):226–229
47. Trope M (1991) Flare-up rate of single-visit endodontics. Int Endod J 24(1):24–26

48. Van Hassel HJ (1971) Physiology of the human dental pulp. Oral Surg Oral Med Oral Pathol 32(1):126–134
49. Vuilleumier PH, Stamer UM, Landau R (2012) Pharmacogenomic considerations in opioid analgesia. Pharmgenomics Pers Med 5:73–87
50. Walton R (2002) Interappointment flare-ups: incidence, related factors, prevention, and management. Endod Top 3:67–76
51. Yesilsoy C, Koren LZ, Morse DR et al (1988) Post-endodontic obturation pain: a comparative evaluation. Quintessence Int 19(6):431–438
52. Young J, Siffleet J, Nikoletti S et al (2006) Use of a behavioural pain scale to assess pain in ventilated, unconscious and/or sedated patients. Intensive Crit Care Nurs 22(1):32–39
53. Yu SM, Bellamy HA, Kogan MD et al (2002) Factors that influence receipt of recommended preventive pediatric health and dental care. Pediatrics 110(6):e73

Local Anesthesia

6

6.1 Depth of Local Anesthesia

Profound anesthesia is the key factor in determining patients' endodontic experience and their assessment of the dentist. Incomplete anesthesia results in pain and increases patient's anxiety with a concomitant drop in their pain threshold. This negative spiral of events affects the patient's endodontic experience and can be prevented. Procedures should be initiated only after profound anesthesia is achieved. Compromising the level of anesthesia is a poor strategy for a clinician hoping to have a satisfied patient.

6.1.1 Soft Tissue and Dental Anesthesia

Soft tissue anesthesia and dental anesthesia must not be confused. A numb lip is often representative of only soft tissue anesthesia or incomplete dental anesthesia rather than profound pulpal anesthesia.

A clinical study determined that patients with lip symptoms following an injection of local anesthesia with a negative response to a cold test were approximately 80 % less likely to experience pain during endodontic treatment compared to those who had only soft tissue signs of anesthesia [9].

Clinical Tips

- Profound Local Anesthesia
- Prior to initiating treatment, the clinician should test the tooth using the chief complaint as a provoking stimulus.
- If the patient's chief complaint is cold sensitivity, a test using Endo-Ice or the equivalent is invaluable in evaluating the depth of anesthesia.
- Similarly, if percussion sensitivity was the primary complaint, that test should be used prior to initiating treatment.

P.A. Rosenberg, *Endodontic Pain*,
DOI 10.1007/978-3-642-54701-0_6, © Springer-Verlag Berlin Heidelberg 2014

- If profound local anesthesia is defined as complete absence of pain, a single injection for a mandibular molar with irreversible pulpitis is usually insufficient.
- A slow inferior alveolar nerve block injection (60 s) results in a higher success rate of pulpal anesthesia than a rapid injection (15 s) [12].

6.2 Anesthesia and Irreversible Pulpitis

Studies in patients with irreversible pulpitis determined that success (mild or no pain upon endodontic access or initial instrumentation) with the inferior alveolar nerve block varied between 15 and 57 % of the time. It is clear that profound anesthesia is often difficult to achieve in patients with irreversible pulpitis with only the INAB. It is often necessary to utilize supplemental injections for these patients [12].

6.3 Anesthetic Failure

A tooth with irreversible pulpitis is significantly more challenging to anesthetize than a normal tooth. There are a number of hypotheses used to explain anesthetic failure and it may be that no single hypothesis explains all clinical situations.

The following hypotheses represent possible causes of anesthetic failure [1]:

- An anesthetic solution may not penetrate to the sensory nerves that innervate the pulp, especially in the mandible.
- The central core theory hypothesizes that nerves on the outside of the nerve bundle supply molar teeth, whereas nerves on the inside supply anterior teeth. Even if deposited at the correct site, anesthetic solution may not diffuse adequately into the nerve trunk to produce an adequate block. This theory may explain elevated anesthetic failure rates in experiments on anterior teeth with inferior alveolar nerve blocks.
- It has been hypothesized that long-term low-level pain may sensitize nociceptors, resulting in a lower pain threshold (allodynia) associated with an exaggerated response to a stimuli (hyperalgesia).
- Basic chemistry postulates that the lowered pH of inflamed tissues reduces the amount of the base form of anesthetic available to penetrate a nerve's membrane. Consequently, there is less of the ionized form within the nerve to achieve anesthesia.
- Although the theory based on pH may have some validity, it is an unlikely cause of anesthesia problems in the mandible. The injection site is distant from the area of inflammation associated with a tooth, and changes in local tissue pH would be unrelated to the anesthesia problem.

- Patients in pain are often apprehensive, which can lower their pain threshold. A negative cycle may occur starting with initial apprehension leading to reduced pain threshold, anesthesia complication, and still further increased apprehension. This can result in a lack of confidence in the dentist.
- The dentist may not allow sufficient time for the anesthetic to diffuse. Onset of complete anesthesia may be slow, particularly with the inferior alveolar block.

6.3.1 Individual Variations

There are significant individual variations among patients and their response to a local anesthetic. Patients may report a history of years of bad experiences with dental anesthesia. It is difficult to ascertain if the problem is due to anatomic factors, a high level of anxiety, or other causes, but the clinician should be prepared to use supplemental techniques. The clinical situation determines the supplemental technique to use.

Clinical Tips

- A patient with irreversible pulpitis and a numb lip and no response to cold testing may still not have complete pulpal anesthesia. Profound lip numbness does not guarantee pulpal anesthesia.
- Pricking the soft tissue with a sharp explorer does not indicate pulpal anesthesia.
- Following an inferior alveolar nerve block, pulpal anesthesia fails in approximately 17 % of first molars, 11 % of first premolars, and 32 % of lateral incisors. All of the patients tested had profound lip numbness [12].
- The onset of lip numbness occurs within 5–9 min.
- Pulpal anesthesia usually occurs within 15–16 min [12].
- Slow onset of pulpal anesthesia occurs after 15 min. In approximately 19–27 % of mandibular teeth, pulpal anesthesia requires more than 15 min. Between 6 and 8 % of patients have onset after 30 min [12].

6.3.2 Supplemental Anesthesia

It is helpful to determine if the patient has a previous history of difficulty in achieving complete local anesthesia. Patients with that history may be more likely to experience continuing anesthetic problems. It is also an indication that supplemental injections may be required.

6.4 Case Selection

Supplemental anesthesia is a critical component of endodontic treatment. Clinicians may vary as to their preferred supplemental approach, but there are some clinical indicators and contraindications to be aware of. It is advised that dentists become proficient in a variety of supplemental injections. Specific clinical factors will dictate, on a case-by-case basis, the most appropriate supplemental injection. For example, deep periodontal pockets would dictate against a ligamental injection.

Another example of case selection for supplemental injections occurs when identifying appropriate cases for an intra-pulpal injection. In cases where there is an anesthesia problem, the intra-pulpal injection is a good choice if there is an existing pulp exposure or near exposure. When a substantial amount of excavation is required prior to the intra-pulpal injection, an alternative supplemental injection should be selected.

Clinical Tips

- Following supplemental injections, it is recommended that all tissue be removed from the canals, in order to avoid problems at the next visit.

6.4.1 Buccal Infiltration

Buccal infiltration injection of articaine after an inferior alveolar nerve block in mandibular first molars without irreversible pulpitis was found to increase anesthetic success. It was determined that a buccal infiltration of 4 % articaine with 1:100,000 epinephrine after an inferior alveolar nerve block significantly increased success (88 %) when compared to using a lidocaine formulation (71 % success). However, for patients with irreversible pulpitis, the supplemental buccal infiltration of articaine was found to be only 58 % successful [12].

Clinical Tips

- Buccal infiltration alone is insufficient for endodontic treatment.
- Mandibular buccal infiltration (and other supplemental injections) should be preceded by an inferior alveolar nerve block and lip symptoms.
- Thick buccal bone in the area of the mandibular second molar may interfere with diffusion of anesthetic during buccal infiltration injections.

6.4.2 Intra-ligamental (PDL) Injection

The periodontal ligament injection (PDL) is a useful injection for posterior teeth after an inferior alveolar nerve block that does not provide profound anesthesia.

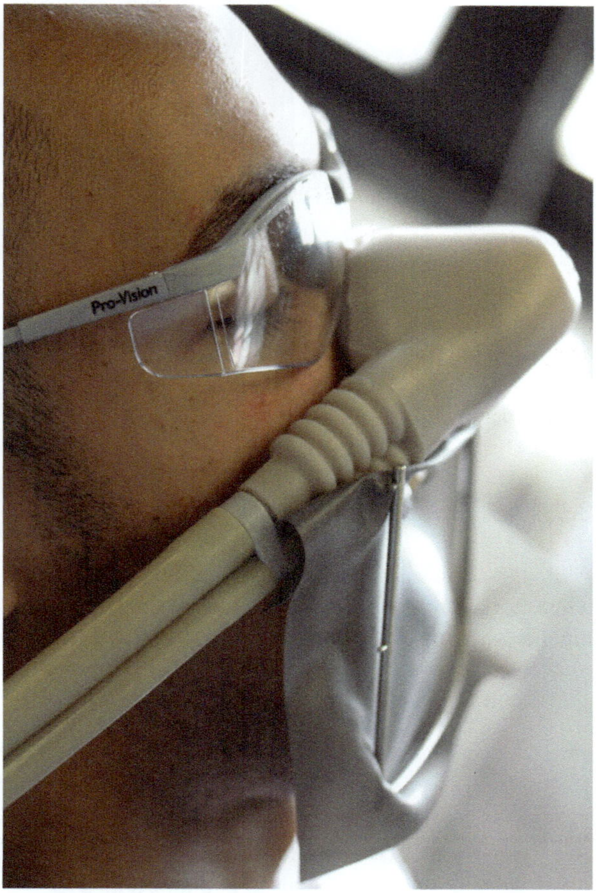

Fig. 6.1 Patient receiving nitrous oxide with rubber dam in place

Back pressure during the injection is an important factor in its success. Absence of back pressure usually leads to failure of the injection [7, 17] (Fig. 6.1).

Special ligamental syringes have not been found to be more effective than a standard syringe [4, 14]. However, the CompuDent CCLAD system (Milestone Scientific Livingston, New Jersey) has been found to increase the duration of anesthesia [2]. It is not uncommon for the patient to experience moderate pain postoperatively following the injection.

The intra-ligamentary injection forces anesthetic solutions through the cribriform plate into the marrow spaces around the tooth [5, 17]. The primary route is not through the periodontal ligament, and the injection may be considered a type of intraosseous injection rather than a pressure injection [7, 17] like intra-pulpal anesthesia.

The intraosseous injection is more successful than the intra-ligamentary injection [13] due to the greater amount of anesthetic solution delivered with the intraosseous injection. However, the intra-ligamentary injection may be helpful if the

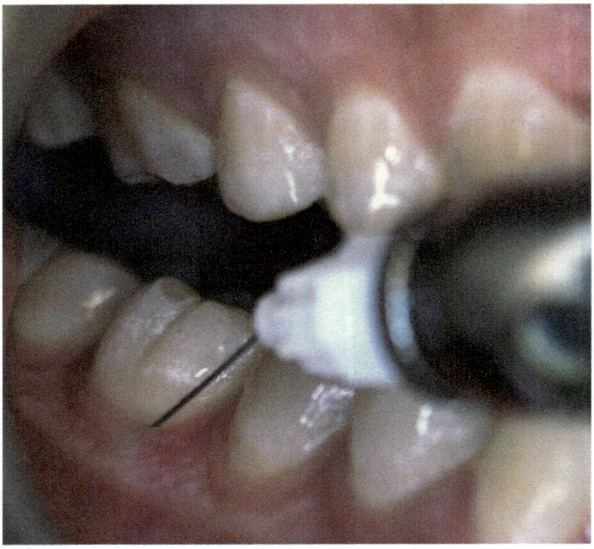

Fig. 6.2 Ligamental injection

clinician is not familiar with the intraosseous injection. A supplemental intra-ligamentary injection is about 75 % successful (Fig. 6.2). Reinjection will increase success to approximately 95 % [10, 11]. However, duration is fairly short when compared to the intraosseous injection.

Clinical Tips

- Intra-ligamentary injections are not recommended in cases of cellulitis, periodontal or endodontic abscesses. It is likely that in these cases, the injection would be painful and unproductive.
- Studies have determined that the most important factor for intra-ligamentary success is back pressure [12].

6.4.3 Intraosseous Injection

The intraosseous injection delivers a local anesthetic solution directly into the cancellous bone adjacent to the tooth to be anesthetized. The addition of the intraosseous injection using 1.8 mL of 2 % lidocaine with 1:100,000 epinephrine after an inferior alveolar nerve block for the first molar provided a rapid onset and a high incidence of pulpal anesthesia (approximately 90 %) for 60 min [12].

The Stabident and X-Tip systems (Fairfax Dental Inc, Miami, FL) are widely used intraosseous systems. The duration of anesthesia is usually sufficient for the complete removal of pulp tissue from the canal(s). At the next visit (if necessary), an inferior alveolar block is usually sufficient.

It should be noted that there is a transient increase in heart rate associated with both systems when injecting epinephrine and levonordefrin-containing anesthetic solutions [12]. Patients may experience a moderate level of pain subsequent to the injection (Fig. 6.3).

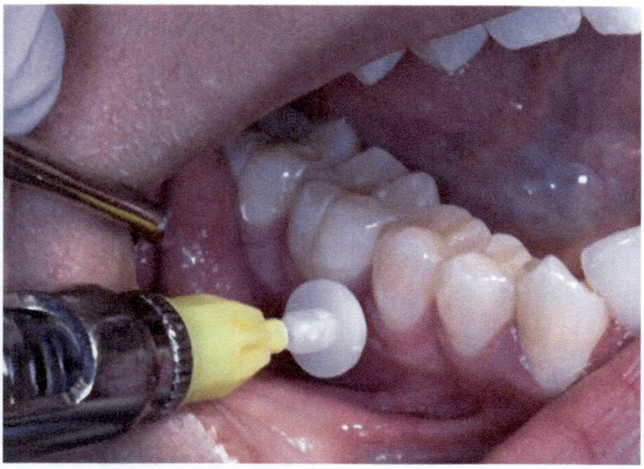

Fig. 6.3 Intraosseous injection. Dentsply Maillefer X-Tip Intraosseous Anesthesia Delivery System

Clinical Tips

- Following inadequate anesthesia, from an inferior alveolar nerve block, the use of an intraosseous injection is an excellent strategy in difficult cases of irreversible pulpitis.

6.4.4 Intra-pulpal Anesthesia

For some teeth, especially mandibular molars with irreversible pulpitis, supplemental injections, even when repeated, do not produce profound anesthesia. This may be an indication for an intra-pulpal injection if there is an existing pulp exposure or near exposure. If extensive excavation is required to reach the pulp, intra-pulpal anesthesia is not recommended since the process would be extremely painful.

The intra-pulpal injection is technique-sensitive and is critically dependent on the establishment of intra-pulpal pressure. Simply flowing an anesthetic into the pulp chamber will be ineffective.

A double-blind randomized clinical study using patients with inadequate local anesthesia determined that intra-pulpal injections of sterile saline or lidocaine 2 % with 1:50,000 epinephrine were both equally effective in producing adequate anesthesia for pulp extirpation [3]. The research demonstrated that an intra-pulpal injection is not true anesthesia. The rapid injection of sterile-distilled water was as effective as an anesthetic solution in creating an "anesthetized" pulp.

It seems that the pressure created in the limited space of the chamber and canal destroys, at least temporarily, the ability of the tissue to transmit impulses. The results of the study, later confirmed by others [16], indicated that the "anesthesia" produced by the intra-pulpal injection is not the result of the anesthetic solution per se. Pressure seemed to be the major factor producing intra-pulpal anesthesia.

If there is a large exposure, the clinician must create pressure by having the needle reach into a canal. The needle should be gently bent at the hub to avoid collapse of the needle under pressure. It is helpful for an assistant to place a hand on the patient's opposite shoulder and massage it. This serves as a momentary

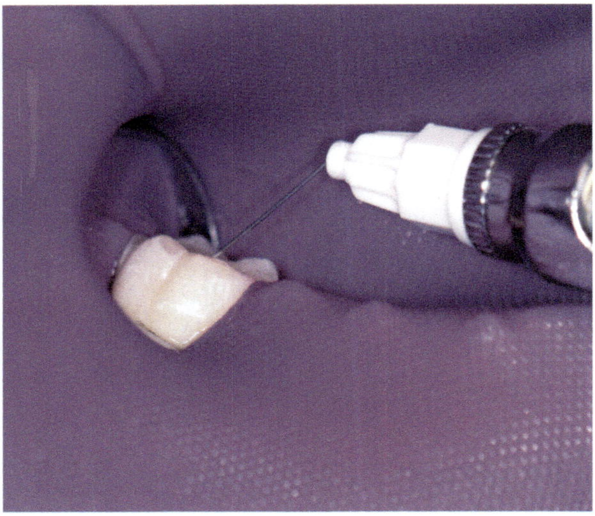

Fig. 6.4 Intra-pulpal injection (Courtesy of Dr. Katsushi Okazaki)

distraction from the pain as the anesthetic is delivered. The dentist should say, while injecting, something like, *"You will feel this for just an instant and then there will be no pain. That's it, that's it…finished."*

This supportive statement and the assistant's involvement are important in solidifying the patient–dentist relationship during a difficult situation. By the time the statement is finished, the injection is completed. Onset of "anesthesia" is virtually immediate and no special syringes or needles are required. The disadvantage of the intra-pulpal technique is that it is painful, but when facing a difficult anesthetic problem, it can save the day (Fig. 6.4).

Clinical Tips

- The use of nitrous oxide in conjunction with the injection is extremely helpful.
- In multi-rooted teeth, each canal may require an intra-pulpal injection.

6.4.5 Nitrous Oxide and Inferior Alveolar Nerve Block

The inferior alveolar nerve (IAN) block is affected by variables including physiological and psychological factors. A high level of patient anxiety can affect success of the inferior alveolar nerve block.

Nitrous oxide has been shown to have both anxiolytic and analgesic properties. A prospective, randomized, double-blind, placebo-controlled study determined the effect of nitrous oxide on anesthetic success of the inferior alveolar nerve block [15].

Patients with symptomatic irreversible pulpitis were randomly assigned to receive an inhalation regime of nitrous oxide/oxygen or room air/oxygen mix (placebo) 5 min before the injection. The success for the inferior alveolar block was 50 % for the nitrous oxide group and 28 % for the placebo group. There was a statistically significant difference between the two groups ($P = .024$) [15].

Clinical Tips

- For the highly anxious patient, the use of nitrous oxide prior to local anesthesia can be of significant value due to its anxiolytic and analgesic properties.

6.5 The "Hot Tooth"

Clinicians treating endodontic patients with a history of symptomatic irreversible pulpitis must be prepared for local anesthetic failures. The term "hot tooth" refers to a tooth that despite all the clinical signs of profound anesthesia remains severely painful as the endodontic procedure is initiated. Although the patient may have a profoundly numb lip and no reaction to an electric pulp tester or to a cold stimulus, there may be severe pain when the dentist starts the access preparation.

This painful problem is associated with treatment of irreversible pulpitis and is frustrating for the patient and dentist. It seems that this scenario occurs most frequently in mandibular molars following a long period of tolerable low-level to moderate pain. Patients who present with a pain of shorter duration seem to be less likely to suffer from this complication. As stated earlier, long-term inflammation has a negative effect on nociceptors (pain receptors). It has been hypothesized that long-term pain may sensitize nociceptors, resulting in a lower pain threshold (allodynia) associated with an exaggerated response to a stimuli (hyperalgesia) .

Clinical Tips

- Administration of nitrous oxide when treating a "hot tooth" can make a major difference in the patient's experience.
- Supplemental anesthetic techniques are often necessary when treating a "hot tooth."

6.5.1 Treatment of the "Hot Tooth"

Following access and establishment of measurement control, it is important to completely remove all tissue from the canal(s). Subsequent visits do not usually involve an anesthetic problem following complete tissue removal.

6.6 Emergency Care

In teeth that respond normally to a local anesthetic, a clinical study demonstrated that *partial pulpectomy* resulted in a higher rate of postoperative pain (13 %) when compared with pulpotomy (6 %). When time does not permit pulpectomy, a pulpotomy, removal of the pulp from the pulp chamber without entering the canal(s), is a highly predictable approach to alleviating pain at an emergency visit [8].

At an emergency visit due to time limitations, it is particularly challenging to remove all tissue and microbial debris from the canal system without pushing toxic material through the periapical foramina into periapical tissues. Establishing an accurate measurement control and maintaining it during instrumentation is critical in avoiding this complication. Instrumenting short of the measurement control results in shredded tissue remnants that can cause postoperative pain and complications. See Chap. 7 for a discussion of endodontic emergencies.

Clinical Tips

- A pulpotomy is a more predictable emergency procedure than is partial instrumentation of canal(s).
- Partial instrumentation results in shredded tissue and can cause increased pain (Figs. 6.5 and 6.6).

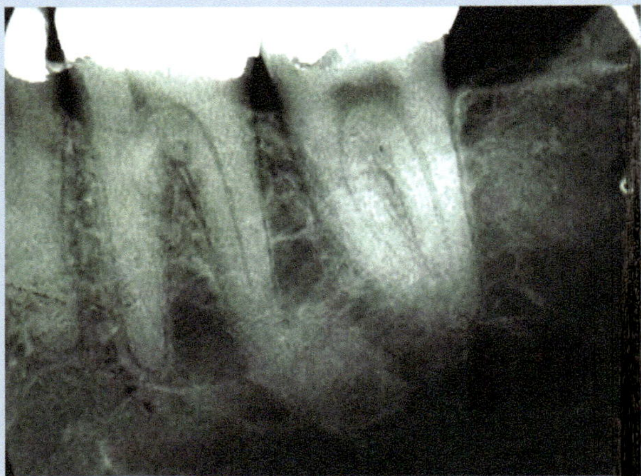

Fig. 6.5 The mandibular left first molar has an apical sclerotic lesion indicating long-term chronic inflammation. The distal portion of the pulp chamber appears calcified. There is evidence of recurrent decay under the distal margin of the crown. Despite these factors, the tooth may have remained asymptomatic for a long period of time. These factors can lead to a "hot tooth" that is difficult to anesthetize

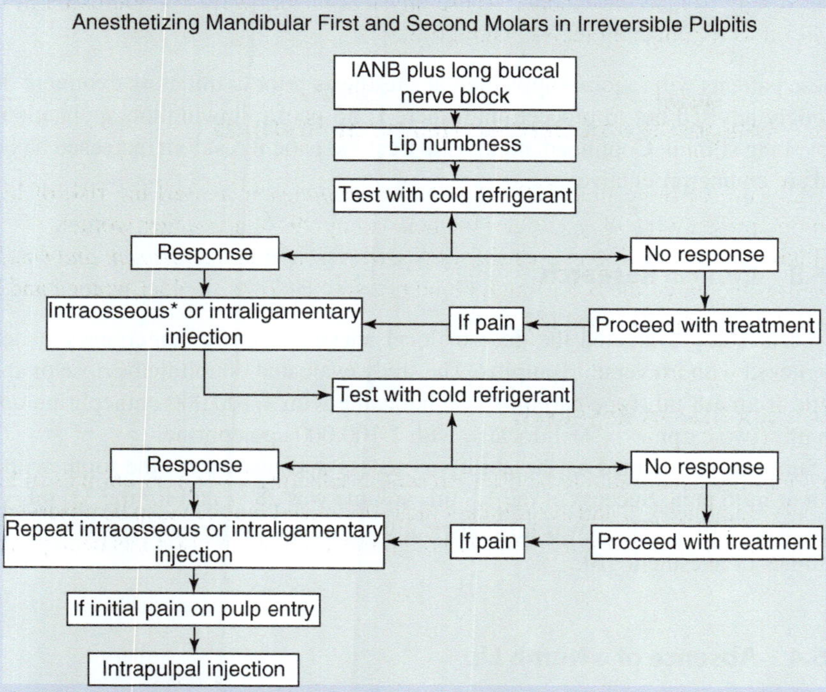

Fig. 6.6 Algorithm for anesthetizing the mandibular first and second molars in irreversible pulpitis. *Before an intraosseous injection, provide a buccal infiltration of 4 % articaine with epinephrine (Reproduced from Reader et al. [12])

6.6.1 Numb Lip and Negative (Painless) Response to Provoking Stimuli

Following an inferior alveolar nerve block, the patient may seem to experience profound anesthesia as evidenced by an extremely numb lip and negative responses to provoking stimuli based on the chief complaint.

However, when endodontic access is started, the patient may still experience acute pain. This frustrating situation points out that the clinician must always be prepared to use a supplemental injection. Despite multiple tests with results indicating complete anesthesia, the patient may still experience pain. The specific supplemental injection should be selected based on the specific clinical situation.

6.6.2 Numb Lip and Positive (Painful) Response to Provoking Stimuli

These patients will require supplemental anesthesia prior to initiating treatment. It is strongly advised not to proceed until there is no pain following the application of provoking stimuli. Continued attempts to treat the patient result in increased anxiety and are counterproductive.

6.6.3 Clinical Research

A recent study evaluated the dose of local anesthetic in 319 emergency patients diagnosed with irreversible pulpitis. The study evaluated doubling the dose of anesthetic from 1.8 mL (one carpule) 2 % lidocaine with 1:100,000 epinephrine up to 3.6 mL (two carpules) 2 % lidocaine with 1:100,000 epinephrine.

Success was defined as the ability to access and instrument the tooth without pain or mild pain. Success of the 1.8 mL volume was 28 % and for the 3.6 mL volume, it was 39 %. There was no statistically significant difference between the two volumes of anesthetic [6].

6.6.4 Absence of a Numb Lip

Patients in this category require another inferior alveolar nerve block. It is most likely that the anesthetic solution has not diffused sufficiently to reach the central core of the nerve bundle or the solution has not been deposited in proximity to the nerve bundle.

Clinical Tips

- Orientation of the needle bevel (away or toward the mandibular ramus) does not affect anesthetic success or failure.
- It is usually not helpful to give an additional inferior alveolar nerve block to a patient with profound lip numbness but still experiences pain during treatment.
- There is good evidence that increasing the volume of anesthesia from one cartridge to two cartridges of lidocaine or increasing the epinephrine concentration from 1:100,000 to 1:50,000 will not provide better pulpal anesthesia.
- A cartridge of either mepivicaine or prilocaine will be as effective for an inferior alveolar nerve block as lidocaine for 50–55 min.
- Clinical trials have failed to demonstrate statistical superiority of articaine over lidocaine for nerve blocks.
- Clinical trials have demonstrated inconsistent findings in comparing articaine's and lidocaine's association with paresthesia [12].

Reversal of Pulpal and Soft Tissue Anesthesia

In a clinical study, Phentolamine significantly ($P<.05$) reduced duration of both pulpal and soft tissue anesthesia when administered at either 30 or 60 min after an inferior alveolar block injection.

It was concluded that Phentolamine would be beneficial for patients who would like to experience a more rapid return to normal soft tissue function and sensation after the administration of local anesthesia. However, because pulpal anesthesia is also reversed fairly rapidly, Phentolamine should be administered at the end of the dental appointment [12].

6.7 Self-Assessment

- A patient has a full crown on a tooth and a chief complaint of pain on cold. Despite a profoundly numb lip and no response to the application of cold, severe pain occurs when the access preparation is started. What should you do?
  A ligamental or intraosseous injection should be used as a supplemental injection. An intra-pulpal injection is not appropriate because there is a substantial amount of tooth structure remaining prior to exposure. Nitrous oxide can be a valuable adjunct.

Clinical Tips

- It is important to note that reversing the effect of a local anesthetic short of its normal duration reduces the valuable postoperative analgesic effect of the anesthetic.

What is the best means of assessing the depth of a patient's anesthesia?

- Test the tooth using the chief complaint as a basis for evaluation of the depth of anesthesia.
- If there was initially thermal sensitivity, retest using a cold or heat stimuli. If there was sensitivity to percussion, retest by percussing the tooth.
- If pain is elicited during retesting, it indicates that anesthesia is not sufficient to start the procedure.

Recommendation An informative and user-friendly book is highly recommended. *Successful Local Anesthesia for Restorative Dentistry and Endodontics,* by Drs. Al Reader, John Nusstein, and Melissa Drum, Quintessence Publishing Co. 2011, provides a wealth of meaningful information concerning local anesthesia.

References

1. American Association of Endodontists, Colleagues for Excellence (2009) Taking the pain out of restorative dentistry and endodontics; current thoughts and treatment options to help patients achieve profound anesthesia
2. Berlin J, Nusstein J, Reader A et al (2005) Efficacy of articaine and lidocaine in a primary intraligamentary injection administered with a computer-controlled local anesthetic delivery system. Oral Surg Oral Med Oral Pathol Oral Radiol Endod 99(3):361–366
3. Birchfield J, Rosenberg PA (1975) Role of the anesthetic solution in intrapulpal anesthesia. J Endod 1(1):26–27
4. D'souza JE, Walton RE, Peterson LC (1987) Periodontal ligament injection: an evaluation of the extent of anesthesia and postinjection discomfort. J Am Dent Assoc 114(3):341–344
5. Dreyer WP, Van Heerden JD, De V Joubert JJ (1983) The route of periodontal ligament injection of local anesthetic solution. J Endod 9(11):471–474
6. Fowler S, Reader A (2013) Is a volume of 3.6 mL better than 1.8 mL for inferior alveolar nerve blocks in patients with symptomatic irreversible pulpitis? J Endod 39(8):970–972
7. Fuhs QM, Walker WA 3rd, Gough RW et al (1983) The periodontal ligament injection: histological effects on the periodontium in dogs. J Endod 9(10):411–415
8. Hasselgren G, Reit C (1989) Emergency pulpotomy: pain relieving effect with and without the use of sedative dressings. J Endod 15(6):254–256
9. Hsiao-Wu GW, Susarla SM, White RR (2007) Use of the cold test as a measure of pulpal anesthesia during endodontic therapy: a randomized, blinded, placebo-controlled clinical trial. J Endod 33(4):406–410
10. Ng YL, Mann V, Gulabivala K (2008) Outcome of secondary root canal treatment: a systematic review of the literature. Int Endod J 41(12):1026–1046
11. Nusstein JM, Reader A, Drum M (2010) Local anesthesia strategies for the patient with a "hot" tooth. Dent Clin North Am 54(2):237–247
12. Reader A, Nusstein J, Drum M (2011) Successful local anesthesia for restorative dentistry and endodontics. Quintessence, Chicago
13. Reisman D, Reader A, Nist R et al (1997) Anesthetic efficacy of the supplemental intraosseous injection of 3 % mepivacaine in irreversible pulpitis. Oral Surg Oral Med Oral Pathol Oral Radiol Endod 84(6):676–682
14. Smith GN, Walton RE, Abbott BJ (1983) Clinical evaluation of periodontal ligament anesthesia using a pressure syringe. J Am Dent Assoc 107(6):953–956
15. Stanley W, Drum M, Nusstein J et al (2012) Effect of nitrous oxide on the efficacy of the inferior alveolar nerve block in patients with symptomatic irreversible pulpitis. J Endod 38(5):565–569
16. Vangheluwe J, Walton R (1997) Intrapulpal injection: factors related to effectiveness. Oral Surg Oral Med Oral Pathol Oral Radiol Endod 83(1):38–40
17. Walton RE (1986) Distribution of solutions with the periodontal ligament injection: clinical, anatomical, and histological evidence. J Endod 12(10):492–500

Flare-Ups

7

7.1 Introduction

Endodontic emergencies are a challenging part of clinical practice. The clinician must have an understanding of inflammatory and infectious processes, pain mechanisms, local anesthesia, the use of therapeutics, and patient management. This chapter will focus on emergencies occurring prior to, during, and after treatment.

As a broad generalization the necrotic tooth (non-vital) represents a microbiological host/parasite challenge, while the vital case represents a problem of managing an inflammatory process in a well-innervated vascular tissue. The unique environment of the pulp is another factor to consider. In both situations, when time permits, removal of the pulp is the initial goal. Swelling, in non-vital cases, may be localized or diffuse. Some swellings may extend through facial plains and be seen as a cellulitis. Each situation requires a somewhat different clinical and pharmacologic strategy based on biological considerations.

The etiology of a flare-up is multifactorial and dependent on interactions between the host's immunological response, infection, and physical damage [5, 28, 36]. An exacerbation (flare-up) has been defined in a number of ways. Some definitions emphasize swelling as being a characteristic symptom while others emphasize the need for an emergency visit. The American Association of Endodontists Endodontic Glossary of Terms 2012 defines a flare-up as, "an acute exacerbation of an asymptomatic pulpal and or periradicular pathosis following the initiation or continuation of root canal treatment."

There are a variety of techniques and therapeutic agents available to treat emergencies. Depending on the circumstances of the emergency, and what we have learned from the best available evidence, clinicians must select the appropriate treatment strategies on a case-by-case basis. Factors such as tooth vitality, the severity of pain and/or swelling, and medical history all have an effect on the strategy and selection of medications.

Prior to determining the course of treatment, the clinician should understand the pathogenesis of the problem. Regardless of when the exacerbation occurs, the goal of treatment is to relieve pain and swelling as quickly as possible.

P.A. Rosenberg, *Endodontic Pain*,
DOI 10.1007/978-3-642-54701-0_7, © Springer-Verlag Berlin Heidelberg 2014

7.2 Incidence of Flare-Ups

As noted earlier, the reported incidence of flare-up varies across studies and ranges from approximately 2 to 20 % of patients, with the higher prevalence generally reported in older studies using classic cleaning and shaping techniques [3, 33, 36]. With such a wide gap in findings, it is likely that differences in research methodologies have had a critical affect on their outcomes.

Investigators examined associations between flare-ups and specific pretreatment factors. Unfortunately, different methodologies and criteria have led to variations in reports of the incidence of flare-ups and significant pretreatment indicators. Using the current American Association of Endodontists (AAE) definition of flare-up, several studies found that a common predisposing clinical condition for the occurrence of a flare-up is a history of preoperative pain. Others noted that an asymptomatic pulp with a periapical lesion was an important factor [3, 5, 32, 33].

Patients with a flare-up usually describe severe pain, swelling, or pressure immediately after anesthesia has dissipated or 1–2 days following treatment. A consistently high incidence of flare-ups should serve as a signal for the clinician to evaluate basic clinical procedures such as accuracy of measurement control and instrumentation. Breakdowns in either of those procedures could account for high rates of exacerbation.

In a prospective clinical study, the level of pain experienced by patients varied from no pain or slight pain up to severe pain. Fifty-seven percent of patients reported no pain after debridement and shaping of the root canal system, although 21 % had slight pain, 15 % had moderate pain, and 7 % had severe pain. Relatively few patients experienced a flare-up or a postoperative problem requiring an unscheduled visit with unplanned treatment intervention to manage the patient's symptoms [36].

7.2.1 Meta-analysis

Meta-analysis is a statistical procedure that integrates the results of several independent studies considered to be combinable. Pooled data from multiple studies increases the sample size and power, thus providing a more precise estimate of a treatment's effect. The decision about whether or not results of individual studies are similar enough to be included in a meta-analysis is a critical issue.

7.2.2 Incidence of Flare-Up

A meta-analysis of the results of previous studies, concerning the incidence of endodontic flare-ups, reviewed all relevant articles published in dental journals in English from 1966 to May 2007. Only six studies met all inclusion criteria. Prospective case series and clinical trials were included in the meta-analysis [34]. The average percentage of incidence of flare-ups for 982 patients was found to be 8.4 %.

Differences in experimental design do not allow for a direct comparison of studies; however, the presence of *preoperative* pain or *mechanical allodynia* (defined as a reduced mechanical pain threshold or percussion sensitivity) was a positive predictor of postoperative pain in more than 15 studies involving more than 6,600 patients [6].

7.3 Predisposing Conditions

When symptomatic pretreatment patients have been included in the study cohort, predisposing conditions include periapical abscess, acute apical periodontitis [31, 32], preoperative pain [21], and swelling. Studies have found that the lowest incidence of flare-ups occurred in patients without periapical pathosis and when a sinus tract is present [32]. It is reasonable to hypothesize that a sinus tract allows drainage and prevents an increase in periapical tissue pressure.

Studies evaluated factors related to postoperative endodontic pain and flare-up. The presence of preoperative pain or mechanical allodynia (reduced mechanical pain threshold or percussion sensitivity) was a significant predictor of postoperative pain in more than 15 studies with a large number of patients [6].

Clinical Tips

- Patients presenting with sensitivity to percussion should be considered at risk for postoperative pain.
- Occlusal reduction in such cases when restorative factors permit can be considered a predictable pain-preventive strategy.

The etiology of a flare-up is multifactorial and dependent on interactions between the host's immunological response, infection, and physical damage. The major causative factor has been described as microbial in origin [32].

There are additional factors that may also predispose a patient to pain. They include genetics, gender, and anxiety. These non-dental factors are being evaluated, and at this time it seems likely that in the future their significance will be more fully understood.

Although no single factor completely predicts the occurrence and severity of postoperative pain, an astute clinician should recognize that the presence of preoperative pain or mechanical allodynia (sensitivity to percussion) is a warning sign that postoperative pain is likely. That warning sign is an indication that pain-preventive steps should be taken. They include preemptive analgesics and occlusal reduction when there is evidence of mechanical allodynia.

7.3.1 Research

A retrospective study analyzed the records of 2,000 patients who had root canal therapy for necrotic teeth. One half of the patients had inter-appointment pain or swelling which required an emergency visit. The other half were patients who reported no complications after cleaning and shaping of their root canals. It was determined that some factors, such as age, sex, tooth type, presence of preoperative pain, presence of allergies, absence of periapical lesions, sinus tract stomas, retreated cases, as well as those receiving prescribed analgesics, had significant effects on the incidence of endodontic inter-appointment emergencies. In contrast, presence of systemic diseases, use of intra-canal medications, and penetration of the foramen with small instruments during length determination had no significant effect on the frequency of these emergencies [32]. The highest incidence of flare-ups was associated with mandibular teeth, retreatment procedures, females over the age of 40, and patients with a history of allergies [32].

7.4 Classic Narratives

At an emergency visit there are classic patient narratives that provide critical information.

Narrative 1

- An example of a classic narrative concerns the patient who describes having had no pain until he/she bit down on something hard which resulted in an immediate sharp lancinating pain and left a tooth tender to even finger pressure. Those few words are a powerful clue as to causation and indicate the need for investigation into a possible vertical or other type of fracture.

Narrative 2

- A patient may report having been awakened at night by pain but feels better as the next day progresses. However, the pain awakens the patient again during the following night but disappears after awakening. This description does not fit the most common profile of irreversible pulpitis. Usually, pulpal pain does not improve as the day goes on.
- This patient would require a differential diagnosis for bruxism, sinusitis, TMD, as well as pain of endodontic origin. Sensibility tests and percussion tests would be important part of the diagnostic process. Normal responses to those tests would prompt the clinician to investigate a non-odontogenic cause of pain (Figs. 7.1 and 7.2).

Clinical Tips

At the emergency visit:

- Patients with a history of long-term low-level pain may pose a problem in achieving profound anesthesia.
- It has been hypothesized that long-term inflammation can sensitize nociceptors resulting in a problem achieving profound anesthesia.
- In these cases clinicians should be prepared to use supplemental anesthetic techniques.

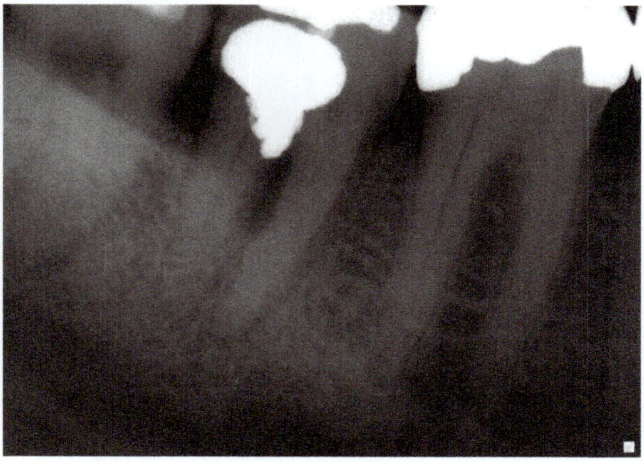

Fig. 7.1 At the emergency visit the initial radiograph indicated that the cause of the patient's pain originated from the mandibular right first molar. However, an additional radiograph including teeth anterior to the molar demonstrated a complicating factor (Courtesy of Dr. Joshua Most)

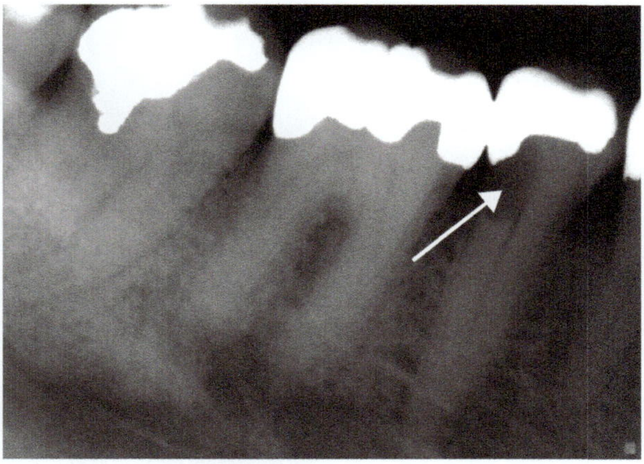

Fig. 7.2 An additional radiograph indicated significant decay under the mandibular right second premolar. *Arrow* points to extensive decay. It was actually this tooth that was the cause of the patient's pain (Courtesy of Dr. Joshua Most)

7.5 Prognosis

At an emergency visit, when the need for endodontic treatment is established, the next consideration is the prognosis and treatment plan. Are there obstacles to satisfactory completion of proposed endodontic therapy? Has root canal therapy been done before? Are there restorative issues? Is there a periodontal component to the case?

Important factors include the following: systemic health of the patient, tooth anatomy, periodontal status, and the ultimate restoration. Is the proposed treatment appropriate for the patient? For example, a patient with poorly maintained dentition may not be a good candidate for root canal treatment, a post and crown.

Economic factors must also be considered. In some countries expenses are paid for by insurance but this is not universal. The goal must be to select the treatment that best serves the patient's overall health needs (Figs 7.3, 7.4, and 7.5).

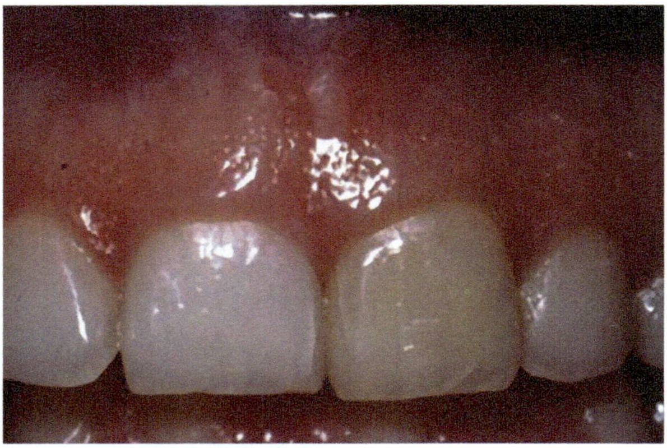

Fig. 7.3 Note difference in color between the central incisors

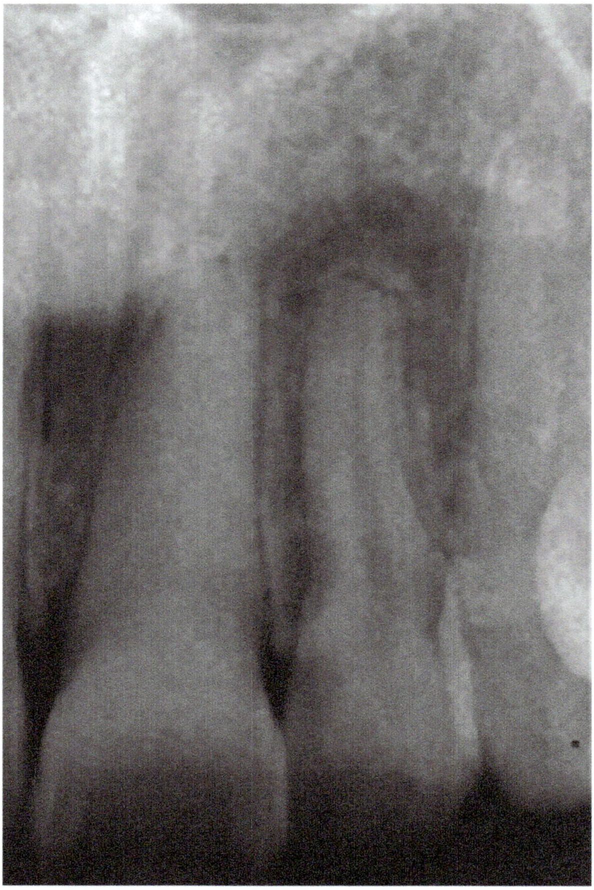

Fig. 7.4 The maxillary left central incisor has extensive diffuse calcification complicating endodontic treatment

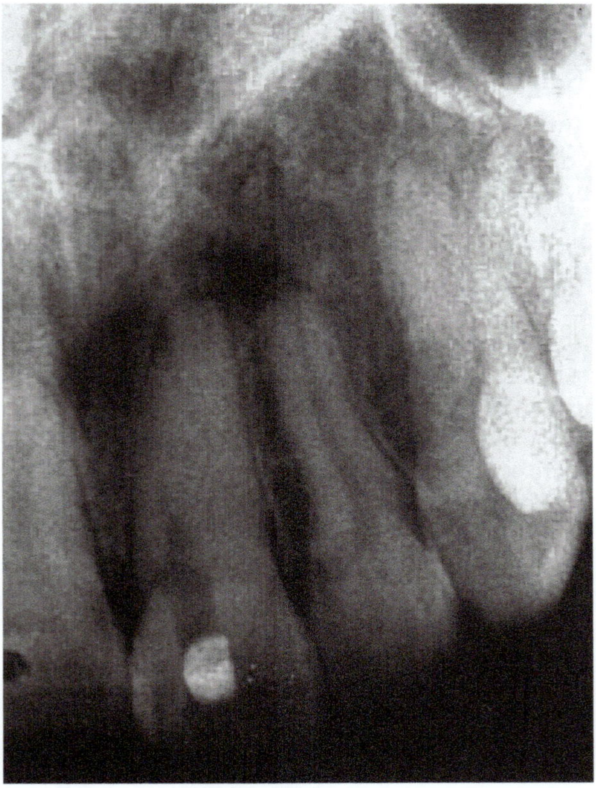

Fig. 7.5 This radiograph taken during an attempt to achieve access indicates that the preparation is not in the canal space and is approaching perforation

7.6 Flare-Up and Outcome

The occurrence of an endodontic flare-up does not appear to influence the long-term prognosis of the tooth. It was reported that the occurrence of flare-ups had no significant influence on the outcome of endodontic treatment when reviewed 8–10 years later [31].

7.7 Causes of Exacerbations During Treatment

Iatrogenic factors associated with exacerbations include incomplete access, inaccurate measurement control, failure to maintain an accurate measurement, failure to completely remove all tissue from the canal, over-instrumentation, and failure to reduce occlusion when it is appropriate.

Clinical Tips

- Establishment of an accurate measurement control is essential in avoiding over-instrumentation and postoperative pain.
- Estimation of measurement increases the likelihood of postoperative pain.
- Use of a rubber stop on instruments is helpful in maintaining measurement.
- During irrigation the needle should not be wedged into the canal or placed close to the apical foramen.
- Irrigate slowly to avoid pushing debris through the periapical foramen.

Non-vital cases differ from vital flare-ups in that even if all iatrogenic factors are addressed, a flare-up may still occur. Necrotic tissue is an ideal site for bacterial colonization and non-vital teeth should be considered to have infected pulps. Pathologic reactions in non-vital cases occur in the periapical tissues due to the extrusion of bacteria and their toxins.

The introduction of oxygen into the canal system upon opening the tooth can upset what may have been a balance between host defensive mechanisms and pathogens. Some anaerobic bacteria may die on exposure to aerobic conditions while other aerobic microbes may proliferate. This may change a chronic asymptomatic case into an acutely painful situation.

Clinical Tips

- Deprived of vascular and neural supply, necrotic pulp tissue provides an excellent culture medium for bacteria.
- Necrotic tissue has neither vascular nor neural supply and is not the source pain during an exacerbation.
- Pain originates from an inflammatory response in the periapical tissues of a tooth with a necrotic pulp.

Pericementitis (inflammation of the periodontal ligament) is a specific symptom often associated with over-instrumentation and/or failure to reduce occlusion when indicated. Pericementitis presents as pain on occlusion and in severe cases pain even on gentle finger pressure against the tooth. When restorative conditions permit, occlusal reduction has been shown to be an effective method of preventing pain due to pericementitis in vital teeth, with any or all of the following indicators: a history of pain, absence of a periapical lesion, and sensitivity to percussion.

In the necrotic case instrumenting significantly short (more than 1–2 mm) of the periapical foramen leaves infected tissue behind that is a focus of bacterial colonization. Instrumenting beyond the foramen results in pushing debris into periapical tissues and causes a marked inflammatory reaction that results in severe pain and swelling. It must be remembered that the painful reaction and/or swelling that occurs in the periapical tissues is caused by bacteria and debris from the canal space being pushed through the periapical foramen. Thus the focus of treatment is eliminating or reducing the bacterial flora in the canal.

7.8 Goal of the Emergency Visit

The goal of an emergency visit is limited to making an accurate diagnosis and bringing the case under control symptomatically. Definitions of what constitutes an endodontic emergency vary but severe pain/swelling is the hallmark of endodontic emergencies.

Traumatic injuries may also be the cause of an emergency visit, but they represent a subset of cases with different considerations than purely endodontic emergencies. It must be noted that some dental traumatic injuries have concomitant injuries to the head and neck that require referral to a physician for evaluation. When doubt exists concerning the need for medical referral, it is wise to favor the referral.

The reader should review textbooks focused on dental trauma for a complete discussion of the subject. A helpful online site providing an extensive source of information concerning trauma is http://www.dentaltraumaguide.org/.

7.9 Managing Emergencies Due to Odontogenic Pain

7.9.1 Emergency Pulpectomy

Definitive non-pharmacologic endodontic treatment includes instrumentation, irrigation, occlusal reduction, and incision for drainage procedures. Numerous studies indicate that definitive treatment alone provides predictable and substantial relief from odontogenic pain. An example of effective treatment is a pulpotomy for patients with irreversible pulpitis. Regardless of the coronal medicament used, it has been reported that a pulpotomy abolished pain in 88 % of patients evaluated 1 day after treatment [7].

When time permits, the most predictable clinical strategy for the treatment of pain of endodontic origin is pulpectomy. Pulpotomy is usually reserved for multi-rooted vital cases when there is insufficient time for a pulpectomy.

7.9.2 Classic Research: Effectiveness of Pulpotomies

Seventy-three teeth with acute irreversible pulpitis had emergency pulpotomies. After removal of the coronal portion of the pulp, sterile cotton pellet or zinc oxide-eugenol cement was placed against the remaining pulp tissue. The cotton pellet was either dry or moistened with camphorated phenol, Cresatin, eugenol, or isotonic saline. This established six different treatment groups following the pulpotomy. All teeth were sealed with zinc oxide-eugenol cement. By means of questionnaires, symptoms were recorded after the anesthetic effect was eliminated and also at 1, 7, and 30 days after treatment. A total of 70 patients (96 %) reported pain relief. Three patients did not experience relief and returned for pulpectomy.

After the first postoperative day, no pain was reported by any of the patients. The frequency of discomfort decreased from 11 % 1 day postoperatively to 1 % 30 days after the emergency treatment. There was no difference in recorded symptoms among the six treatment groups. Thus, removal of caries, pulpotomy, and sealing of the cavity apparently were reliable means to relieve pain. The use of the various dressings did not contribute to the relief of pain [7].

A common question:

- *When instrumenting, should I use 21 or 25 mm hand files instruments?*

  As a general statement, use the instrument closest in length to the measurement. This facilitates maintaining measurement since the handle can serve as a measurement guide. If the measurement is 19, 20, or 21 mm (or shorter), use 21 mm instruments. If the measurement is 23, 24, or 25 mm, use 25 mm instruments. An exception, in some cases, proximity of the file's handle to the occlusal surface, could interfere with electronic apex locators.

7.9.3 Diagnostic Questions and Exacerbations

There are specific questions that a clinician must consider in order to determine the cause of a patient's postoperative pain/swelling and/or pericementitis. Answers to the following questions provide critical information for the clinician enabling him/her to determine the appropriate course of treatment.

- Was the measurement control accurate?
- Was it maintained during instrumentation?
- Was the canal completely instrumented?
- Was the occlusion appropriately reduced if the case fit the prerequisites?
- If there is swelling, is it circumscribed or extensive and spreading through facial planes resulting in cellulitis?
- Is the swelling fluctuant?

7.9.4 Cleaning/Shaping and Irrigation

Cleaning/shaping and irrigation (with sodium hypochlorite) are the basic means of reversing inflammatory and/or infectious processes in the root canal system. Whether or not the pulp is inflamed or infected, it is damaged pulp tissue that is the driving force of endodontic pathosis. As the inflammatory and infectious process progresses, the ultimate end point is devitalization (necrosis) of the pulp and periapical pathosis.

Clinical Tips

- The pathologic process leading to periapical pathosis may occur with or without pain and can be a rapid or insidious process.
- Radiographs give no indication of the patient's symptoms or what is happening at a cellular level.
- In vital cases the goal is to totally remove inflamed well-innervated tissue without causing additional pain. In non-vital cases the focus is on removing microbes and their products from the canal system.

7.9.5 Occlusal Reduction

A number of clinical studies have evaluated the pain-preventive value of occlusal reduction. It is difficult to compare their results of the trials due to different methodologies, inclusion and exclusion requirements, and specific purposes of the study.

A large clinical study investigated the following questions: "Are there specific clinical findings that indicate a need for occlusal reduction? Can a reliable clinical profile be developed of patients most likely to benefit from occlusal reduction?" [27].

The research hypothesized that there may be specific preoperative conditions that are statistically significant indicators for occlusal reduction following instrumentation. This approach varied from previous research that placed all endodontic cases together in a single group without accounting for the importance of clinical variables. The earlier studies also had a smaller sample size.

Among the conditions evaluated were the presence or absence of pulp vitality, preoperative pain, and percussion sensitivity; presence of a periapical radiolucency, a stoma, and swelling; and a history of bruxism. The purpose of the study was to evaluate specific clinical factors as indicators for occlusal reduction following endodontic instrumentation.

A statistically valid profile of patients most likely to benefit from occlusal reduction was developed. In that study of 117 patients [27], approximately twice as many patients (80 %) with a diagnosis of irreversible pulpitis, who underwent occlusal reduction, reported no posttreatment pain when compared to no occlusal reduction control subjects.

Research Findings

Occlusal reduction was found to result in the prevention of postoperative pain when any or all of the following indicators were present:

- Sensitivity to percussion
- Vital tooth
- History of pain
- Absence of a periapical radiographic lesion

Interestingly, even when all of those pain predictors were present, occlusal reduction resulted in the complete absence of postoperative pain. This remarkable result is likely due to relieving occlusal stress from the periodontal ligament [27].

Biology: Occlusal Reduction

- A possible biological explanation for the effect of occlusal reduction came from a study that examined pulp and periodontal ligament samples taken from 28 healthy premolars to be extracted for orthodontic reasons. One half of the teeth had a resin block over their occlusal surfaces and patients chewed gum for 30 min. The remaining patients had no occlusal interference and also chewed gum for 30 min. They found that occlusal trauma, experimentally induced, markedly increased expression of substance P, a pro-inflammatory mediator, in the pulp and periodontal ligament [4].

- That research finding represents a possible biological explanation for what happens to the periodontal ligament when a tooth is either high in occlusion or taken out of occlusion. Occlusal reduction represents an important pain-preventive strategy in the presence of specific indicators [4].

Recent Research

A recent prospective clinical examination investigated the probability of the incidence, intensity, duration, and triggering of post-endodontic pain. The study considered factors related to the patient (age, gender medical evaluation) and to the affected tooth's location, number of canals, pulp vitality, preoperative pain, periapical radiolucency, previous emergency access, and presence of opposing occlusal contacts [2].

A total of 500 single-visit root canal treatments were performed on patients referred to an endodontist. Shaping of root canals was performed manually, and apical patency was maintained with a size 10 K file. A 5 % sodium hypochlorite (NaOCl) solution was used for irrigation. Canals were filled using gutta-percha and AH-Plus sealer with lateral compaction. Independent factors were recorded during treatment, and characteristics of post-endodontic pain (incidence, intensity, type, and duration) were later surveyed through questionnaires.

Findings of Predictive Models

- It was determined that the incidence of post-endodontic pain was significantly lower when the treated tooth was not a molar ($P=0.003$), demonstrated periapical radiolucency ($P=0.003$), had no history of previous pain ($P=0.006$) or emergency endodontic treatment ($P=0.045$), and had no occlusal contacts ($P<0.0001$).
- The probability of experiencing moderate or severe pain was higher with increasing age ($P=0.09$) and in mandibular teeth ($P=0.045$). The probability of pain lasting more than 2 days was increased with age ($P=0.1$) and decreased in males ($P=0.007$) and when a radiolucent lesion was present on radiographs ($P=0.1$) [2].

Order of Importance

It was determined that the probability of developing post-endodontic pain depended on the following factors in order of importance:

- Presence of occlusal contacts
- Presence of preoperative pain
- Presence of radiolucency
- Tooth type
- Presence of previous emergency endodontic treatment

Duration of Pain

- The duration of post-endodontic pain was predicted by factors: age, gender, and the presence of radiolucency. The findings are similar to previously reported results [27]. It was also demonstrated that preoperative pain was a good predictor of the incidence but not of the intensity of post-endodontic pain [2].

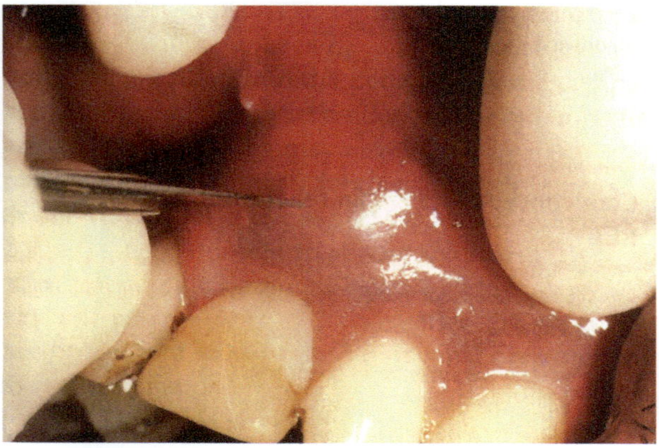

Fig. 7.6 Incision in an attempt to establish drainage from a fluctuant swelling

Intensity of Pain

- The intensity of post-endodontic pain depended on the type of the tooth and the age of the patient [2].

In contrast, through the use of statistical analyses, other authors reported that the intensity of preoperative pain is related to the intensity of post-endodontic pain [32], and that patients experiencing moderate or severe preoperative pain were five times more likely to have this same level of pain after the treatment as compared to patients with mild or no preoperative pain [21].

7.9.6 Incision and Drainage (I&D)

When there is significant fluctuant swelling, incision and drainage is recommended following cleaning/shaping and irrigation. The goal of I&D is to evacuate an exudate (pus) from the periapical tissues. The result is reduced periapical tissue pressure and a reduction in the patient's pain due to distended tissue.

Instrumentation, irrigation, dressing, and closure are all important in eliminating or reducing the level of contaminants in the canal. Those procedures prevent further bacterial penetration from the canal space that would result in continued periapical inflammation. Dressing and closure of the tooth should be accomplished as soon as active drainage stops, which may take several minutes. When indicated, systemic antibiotics can be expected to be more effective following canal instrumentation, irrigation, dressing, and closure.

Antibiotics should not be used without concomitant cleaning/shaping and irrigation and are never indicated as a treatment for pain. The removal of dead lymphocytes and dead bacteria from an infectious site can bring more rapid resolution of symptoms and prevent extension of the infectious process. Return of local vascular flow is important in reaching and maintaining systemic antibiotic levels, as well as reducing local tissue acidity, thus enhancing action of local anesthetics when an infiltration injection is used (Figs. 7.6 and 7.7).

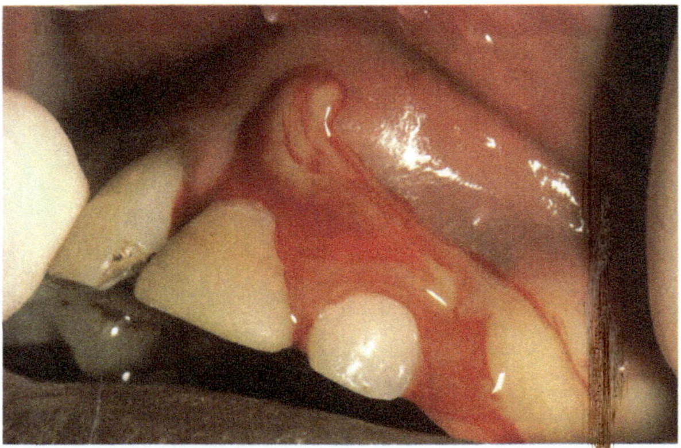

Fig. 7.7 Drainage established following the incision

Clinical Tips

- Prior to incision and drainage (I&D), it is important to instrument and irrigate the canal(s) and place an antimicrobial dressing in order to reduce microbiological factors originating in the canal system.
- Antibiotics should not be used without concurrent cleaning/shaping and irrigation.
- It is important to see the patient 24–48 h after an incision and drainage procedure for re-cleaning/shaping and irrigation.

7.9.7 Anesthetic Injections in the Presence of Swelling

Injecting local anesthetic into a swollen area is contraindicated. The reasons include possible spread of infection, ineffective anesthesia due to reduced pH, and pain associated with the injection. However, a study found that local anesthetics could be successfully used in inflamed tissues despite being acidified [35].

The primary reason for not injecting into an area of swelling is that it is extremely painful and usually relatively ineffective. Increased blood supply associated with the swelling results in the anesthetic solution being carried away into the systemic circulation rather than causing profound anesthesia with good duration. However, injecting at the periphery of a swelling usually provides sufficient local anesthesia for an incision and drainage procedure.

7.9.8 Drainage and Sinus Tracts

Chronic drainage through a sinus tract reduces the occurrence of flare-ups because it provides ongoing drainage for apical tissues due to bacteria in the canal system.

In cases of acute exacerbation of a chronic periapical lesion or a posttreatment endodontic abscess, establishing drainage through the oral mucosa provides effective emergency management. The rationale for an incision and drainage (I&D) procedure is to facilitate the evacuation of pus, microorganisms, and toxic products from the periapical tissues [28]. This is especially important when drainage cannot be established through the root canal. I&D results in decompression of periapical tissue pressure and usually provides significant pain relief.

7.9.9 Abscess After Obturation

Assuming, the root canal filling appears to be satisfactory, but an abscess occurs shortly after obturation, incision and drainage of the fluctuant tissue is an important emergency procedure. In cases of inadequately filled canals, in addition to incision and drainage, the filling material should be removed in order to allow for additional drainage through the root canal space and re-cleaning/shaping and irrigation. Antibiotics are usually not indicated in cases of a localized swelling but can be used to supplement clinical procedures in cases where there is poor drainage and if the patient has a concomitant trismus, cellulitis, fever, or lymphadenopathy.

7.9.10 Trephination

Trephination is a clinical technique that has been suggested to reduce intraosseous pressure. Cortical trephination is defined as the surgical perforation of the alveolar bone in an attempt to release accumulated periradicular tissue exudate. Studies have evaluated the effectiveness of cortical trephination to prevent and/or relieve post-treatment pain [26].

Although trephination has been advocated as a means of reducing pain during or after endodontic therapy, several randomized clinical trials have failed to demonstrate a significant difference between the effect of trephination with pulpectomy and the effect of pulpectomy alone [9, 15, 18].

A study compared the difference in postoperative pain relief in patients with acute periradicular pain of pulpal origin when treated by either pulpectomy alone or pulpectomy with cortical trephination. There were no significant differences between the groups.

Another study performed a randomized blinded study to evaluate postoperative pain and swelling after performing trephination in symptomatic teeth with periradicular radiolucent lesions. They also found no significant reduction in pain or swelling in the trephination group. There appears to be no significant benefit from cortical trephination procedures [26].

However, there are some clinicians who advocate trephination in cases of persistent pain during endodontic treatment that is not relieved by instrumentation, irrigation, and medication. The window created in overlying bone is thought to decompress the area thus providing relief from the persistent pain [28]. If the clinician decides to opt for trephination, the procedure should be done in conjunction with an appropriate flap and identification of the root apex. Estimating the location of the apex can result in inadvertent damage to the wrong tooth.

Clinical Tips

Prophylactic antibiotics

- Prophylactic antibiotics have been shown to be ineffective in the prevention of flare-ups. This has been established in a series of prospective, randomized, double-blind, placebo-controlled clinical trials that found prophylactic antibiotics (penicillin or amoxicillin) to be ineffective in preventing posttreatment flare-ups in cases of pulp necrosis with periapical lesions in asymptomatic [22] and symptomatic [8] teeth as well as in untreated teeth with irreversible pulpitis [17].

7.10 Procedural Accidents

A procedural accident often impedes therapy or makes it impossible for therapy to be completed. An example of such a procedural accident occurs following instrument separation (breakage). The result may be an inability to complete instrumentation or place an adequate root canal filling. At times, the separated instrument can be removed or bypassed, but often it forms an obstacle to further treatment. The risk of endodontic failure increases particularly when a procedural accident occurs during treatment of an infected tooth. Important variables affecting the outcome, following instrument separation, include the location of the separated instrument and whether or not the cleaning/shaping and irrigation was completed at the time of separation. Endodontic procedural errors are not usually the direct cause of treatment failure. They do increase the risk of failure because of the clinician's inability to eliminate tissue debris and microorganisms from infected root canals [11, 12].

Clinical Tips

- Irrigating solutions, intra-canal dressings, and sealers can cause pain when extruded through the periapical foramen into the periapical tissues.

7.10.1 Sodium Hypochlorite Accident

Although sodium hypochlorite is widely used because of its bactericidal and tissue dissolving properties, its misuse can have serious outcomes. A sodium hypochlorite accident refers to extrusion of sodium hypochlorite through the periapical foramen. It immediately results in severe pain, swelling, and ecchymosis of the mucous membranes and face. In most cases, the symptoms usually disappear within in 7–14 days.

Clinical Tips

- Sodium hypochlorite accidents can be prevented.
- The solution should be delivered slowly and the needle not wedged in the canal.
- Especially in cases with an open apex, the needle should be placed some distance from the apical foramen.
- Treatment is based on supportive therapy including antibiotics and analgesics (Figs. 7.8, 7.9, 7.10, and 7.11).

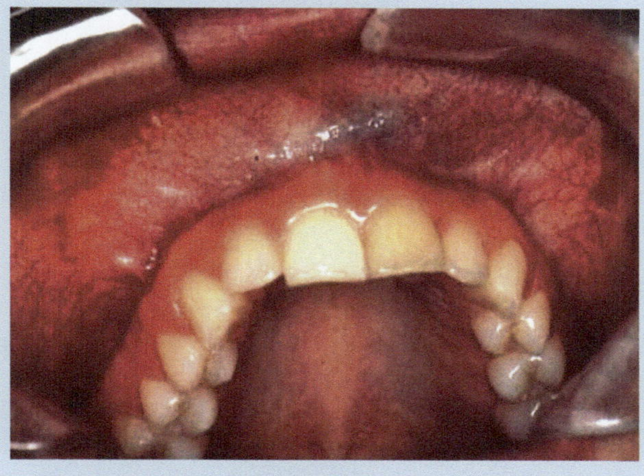

Fig. 7.8 Immediate soft tissue response to NaOCl irrigation. Note edema and hemorrhagic response. The patient experienced severe pain

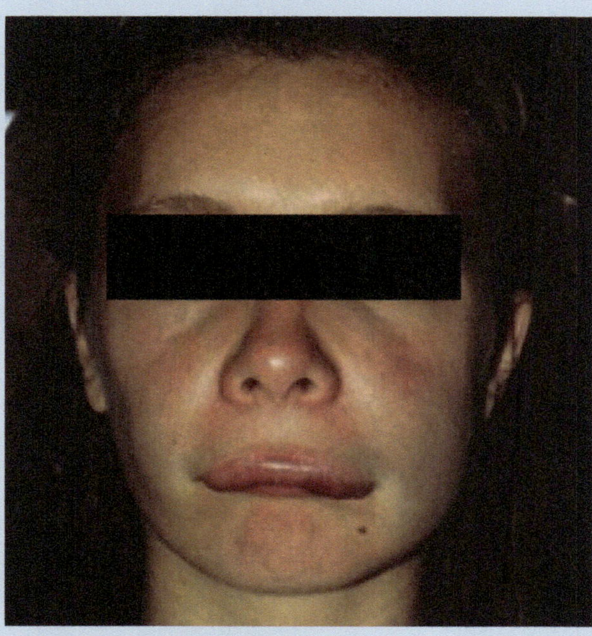

Fig. 7.9 Facial swelling immediately following the NaOCl accident

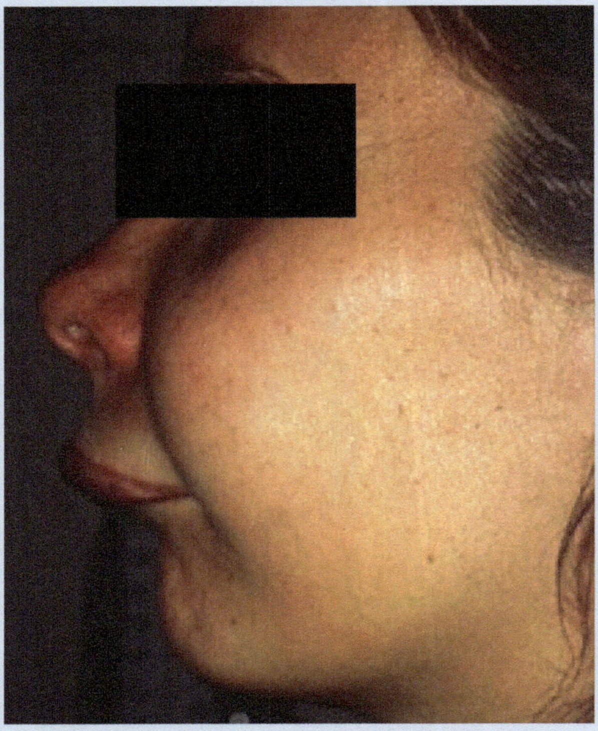

Fig. 7.10 Profile of patient immediately following the NaOCl accident

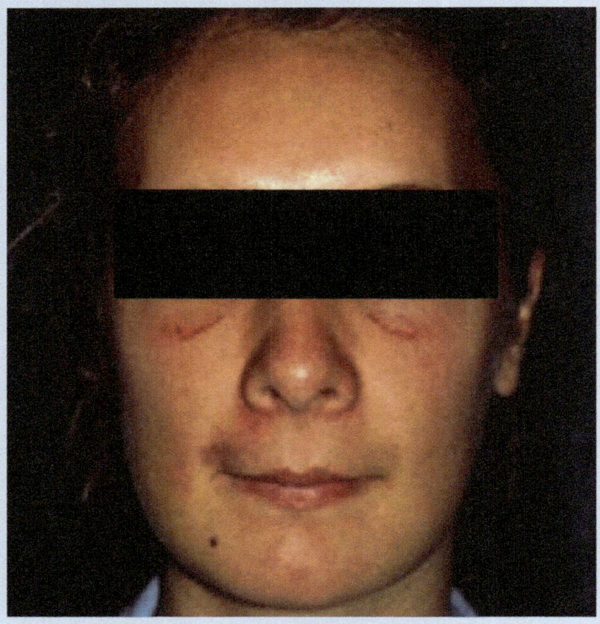

Fig. 7.11 One week after the NaOCl accident

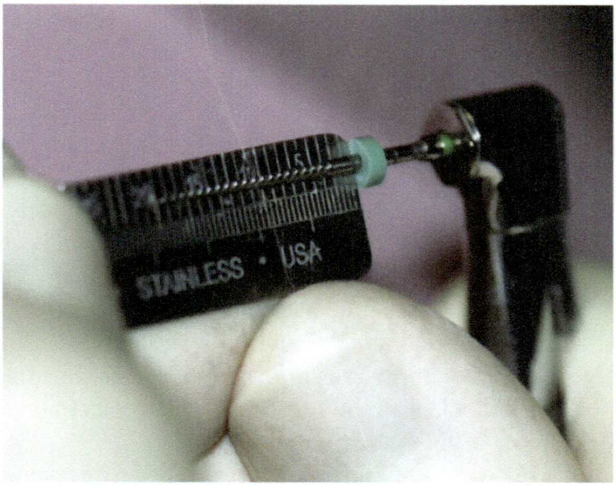

Fig. 7.12 A measurement control using a millimeter ruler

7.10.2 Inadequate Access

Inadequate access predisposes the case to complications. If the chamber is not fully uncovered, canal orifices in multi-rooted teeth may not be identified. This results in pulp tissue being left behind causing persistent pain and potential for bacterial colonization.

Instruments forced to bend under cusps in order to enter canals are prone to separation when stressed by canal curvatures. The goal of access is to uncover all canals and allow straight-line access to canals. If access is incomplete, tissue may remain in the chamber and serve as an area of bacterial colonization resulting in pain.

7.10.3 Establishing Measurement Control

In some areas, anatomic structures, like the maxillary sinus, may prevent an accurate reading of a measurement radiograph. Severe gaggers may not be able to tolerate a radiograph and for pregnant patients, radiographs should be minimized. In those situations, an apex locator should be the used to determine an accurate measurement. The goal is to establish a measurement approximately 1 millimeter (mm.) short of the radiographic apex and maintain it during instrumentation.

An advantage of a measurement radiograph is that it provides important information beyond the measurement. Additional roots, periodontal defects, and anatomic variations may be seen that were not seen on the initial radiographs. In contrast, an apex locator provides only a number and no further information (Fig. 7.12).

Both radiographs and apex locators are technique sensitive. When using an apex locator, it is suggested that excessive irrigating solution and/or blood be eliminated prior to its use. Following the initial measurement reading, the instrument should be removed from the canal and then reinserted in order to validate the initial measurement. Inconsistent readings may be due to open apices, contact of the instrument with a metal restoration, excessive fluid in the canal, or contamination with canal lubricants.

7.10.4 Radiographs

Clinical Tips

- A slight increase (+5°) in vertical angulation results in a sharper image of the apical third of the root.
- Radiographs of maxillary premolars should be taken slightly from the mesial in order to separate buccal and palatal canals.
- Radiographs of mandibular molars should be taken slightly from the mesial in order to separate mesiobuccal and mesiolingual canals.
- When a radiograph is taken from the mesial, the mesiobuccal canal of a mandibular molar is thrown to the distal. In a maxillary pre molar a radiograph taken slightly from the mesial causes the buccal canal to be visualized distal to the palatal canal.
- In order to minimize radiation, take the measurement radiograph of multirooted teeth with all instruments in place and always use a lead shield and thyroid collar for the patient.
- It is useful to use magnification when viewing radiographs.
- Establish a reference point on the tooth (incisal edge or mesiobuccal cusp) and record measurements in millimeters.
- Avoid estimation when an instrument is more or less than 1 mm short or long of the root apex. The greater the estimation, the more likely it is that an error will occur and result in pain.

7.10.5 Maintaining Measurement Control

Maintaining measurement control while instrumenting is an essential component of a pain-preventive strategy. Some instruments have marks on their shafts indicating the length. This is useful for the clinician focused on maintaining an accurate measurement. A rubber stop appropriately placed is also helpful in maintaining measurement control.

Instrumenting short of the measurement control increases the risk if leaving shredded tissue in the canal that is a cause of postoperative pain and a potential source of infection. Instrumenting past the apical foramen results in inflammation of apical tissues resulting in pain.

Clinical Tips

- Instrumenting short of the measurement control complicates filling the root canal. It is frustrating to find that the master gutta-percha cone seems to be well fit but remains 3–5 mm short of the original measurement. This common problem results from a failure to maintain the measurement during instrumentation and results in ledge formation.
- The best strategy to address this problem is to re-instrument starting with smaller hand files. It is advisable to bend the last millimeter or two of the file at a 45° angle, in an attempt to reestablish the correct measurement.

7.10.6 Instrumentation and Flare-Ups

Inter-appointment flare-ups most often follow instrumentation of the canal system. The biological factors resulting in pain in cases with irreversible pulpitis (vital cases) and pain/swelling in necrotic (non-vital) cases may differ and will be reviewed.

Most importantly, before emergency treatment is initiated, the clinician should understand the biological cause of the problem. For example, was there an iatrogenic component to the exacerbation, as occurs when an inaccurate measurement is used or an accurate measurement was established but not maintained?

The vital flare-up may be caused by shredded tissue in the root canal or from inflammation of periapical tissues due to over-instrumentation or excess root canal filling. Another possibility concerns the tooth's occlusion. Was the tooth left in occlusion despite indications to the contrary? This would further exacerbate an inflamed periodontal ligament resulting in pericementitis.

There are significant biological differences in vital and non-vital exacerbations. As stated earlier, the challenge for a clinician while treating a vital tooth is essentially focused on removing well-innervated inflamed tissue from a complex canal system without causing additional inflammation and pain. The vital flare-up may be caused by shredded tissue in the root canal or from inflammation of periapical tissues due to over-instrumentation or excess root canal filling.

Biologically, the non-vital (necrotic) case poses a different challenge. Here the issue for the clinician is the presence of microbes in necrotic tissue. These microbes can be a mix of aerobic and anaerobic species of varying degrees of virulence and cause defensive inflammatory and immune reactions, which result in pain and swelling. The primary challenge is to avoid pushing infected material from the root canal system into the periapical tissues during instrumentation.

It is important to remember that in necrotic cases the reaction causing pain and or swelling is taking place in the periapical tissues and not the root canal. In an exacerbating non-vital case, a patient may complain of tooth pain, but in reality the pain is coming from inflammation and mediator release in the periapical tissues and bone. In non-vital cases, the root canal no longer contains a viable neural or vascular supply.

7.11 Other Factors Predisposing Patients to Pain

There is an increasing body of evidence indicating that there may be additional factors predisposing patients to pain. These variables may influence healing and the response of patients to analgesics. The factors include genetics, gender, and level of anxiety. Other comorbidities to be considered include social/environmental factors, patient compliance, and pharmacodynamics. Some factors are readily apparent (e.g., patient's gender), while others (patient's genetics) are unknown to the clinician. The role of anxiety in the pain process is reviewed in Chap. 4.

A review of those variables will broaden the clinician's appreciation of variables that are often not considered in searching for the cause of pain. The factors may help to explain why one patient has a smooth postoperative course, while another has severe pain and does not react well to an analgesic. Of course, iatrogenic factors are always a potential cause of pain but other variables, not always fully appreciated, may be contributing factors. There is increasing evidence that other factors including genetics, gender, and anxiety may predispose a patient to pain.

7.11.1 Genetics

It is increasingly common to find genetic studies in the endodontic literature. Although these studies represent the early stages of investigating endodontic/genetic relationships, it seems evident that the investigatory process will continue and expand. The answers to some of our biological questions including abscess formation, healing or failure to heal, and effectiveness of specific pharmacologic agents may depend, at least in part, on a patient's genetic makeup. It is interesting to imagine what possibilities exist in the future of endodontics as knowledge of genetics expands.

One study suggested that genetic factors may be associated with a susceptibility to develop symptomatic dental abscesses. Another report suggested that some genetic factors might influence a patient's response to endodontic treatment of teeth with apical periodontitis [30].

Other findings suggested that specific genetic markers associated with increased pro-inflammatory IL-1B (a key regulator of host response) could contribute to increased susceptibility to periapical pathosis [16]. Additionally, a study suggested that a genetic predisposition can contribute to persistent apical periodontitis [13].

These studies and others point the way to the possibility of a complex mix of factors involved in endodontic pain and treatment outcome.

7.12 Diagnostic Questions and Exacerbations

Several diagnostic questions are important for the clinician to consider when confronted with pain/swelling or pericementitis. Answers to these questions provide critical information for the clinician considering the appropriate course of treatment.

- Was the measurement control accurate?
- Was it maintained during instrumentation?
- Was the canal completely instrumented?
- Was the occlusion appropriately reduced if the case fit the prerequisites?
- Is there swelling present?
- If there is swelling, is it circumscribed or extensive and spreading through facial planes resulting in cellulitis?
- Is the swelling fluctuant?

7.13 Post-obturation Emergencies

A histologic study showed that the most favorable response of periapical tissues occurred when both instrumentation and filling were short of the periapical constriction [24]. A clinical study found that the best treatment outcome in infected teeth with periapical lesions occurred when the periapical terminus of the filling was 0–2 mm short of the radiographic apex [31]. The same study determined that the prognosis was decreased with either significant under fill or over fill. These findings have been corroborated by other research reports.

Post-obturation emergencies may include pain and/or diffuse swelling. At the start of the filling visit, tenderness to palpation or to percussion, or an inability to comfortably bite on the tooth, is a predictor of post-obturation pain. In such cases, it is strongly recommended to defer obturation until the patient is pain-free and the tooth can be used in function. When teeth are obturated despite the presence of pericementitis, postoperative pain is the likely outcome.

7.13.1 Questions Concerning Post-obturation Exacerbations

- Was the patient symptomatic prior to obturation?
  Pain prior to filling predisposes the patient to post-obturation pain.
- If there is swelling, is it localized or diffuse and fluctuant?
  Swelling is an indicator of infection.
- Is the tooth overfilled?
  Overfilling can cause a foreign body reaction.
- Is the pain/swelling increasing?
  Increasing pain/swelling is a sign of infection.

7.13.2 Should I Remove the Filling?

During treatment of an exacerbation following filling the clinician must decide whether or not it is necessary to remove the root canal filling(s). Much depends on the condition of the tooth prior to obturation and the quality of the filling. Was the tooth asymptomatic or did symptoms persist following instrumentation? Filling canals in the presence of continuing symptoms is a predictor of post-obturation complications.

The nature of the swelling should also be considered. If there is swelling, is it localized or fluctuant? The type of swelling influences the treatment. Fluctuant swellings can be treated by incision and drainage with supplementary antibiotics. Non-fluctuant swellings are not appropriate for incision and drainage and may be treated with antibiotics if the filling is to be maintained.

Treatment for necrotic post-obturation exacerbations may range from using pharmaco-therapeutics including analgesics and/or antibiotics up to retreatment with or without incision for drainage. Antibiotics should not be used in vital cases.

The clinician must consider the variables and then determine if the primary cause of the patient's symptoms is inflammatory in nature, due to the procedure, or active infection. In most cases, if basic endodontic principles have been followed, and if the root canal filling is of good quality, it does not have to be removed.

7.13.3 Gross Overfilling

It is well established that overfilling results in delayed healing and ultimately a lower success rate than fillings that are flushed to the end of the root or a millimeter or two within the root. Overfillings result in an inflammatory foreign body reaction that can cause prolonged pain and tenderness in the muco-buccal fold adjacent to the root apices.

There are several factors often involved resulting in gross overfilling. For example, open apex cases or those with unusually large apical openings are prime candidates for overfilling. Good initial radiographs can provide the clinician with a warning, in advance of treatment, of the potential for overfilling. This information should impact the instrumentation of the canal as well as cone selection and the filling process. During instrumentation of such canals, the clinician should attempt to maintain apical anatomy and not unnecessarily enlarge that area.

Gross overfilling can be the cause of prolonged pain and have serious consequences if the mandibular canal or maxillary sinus is involved. Attempting to remove grossly overfilled gutta-percha by instrumenting through the end of the root may compound the damage. The decision concerning what is best for the patient following gross overfilling depends on local anatomy, amount of overfilling and the overall treatment plan.

Prompt consultation on a case-by case basis is highly recommended. If the maxillary sinus or mandibular canal is not impacted by the overfill, periodic reevaluation of the case may be a reasonable approach since absorption of the excess filling is a common occurrence.

Mandibular Canal

Gutta-percha or sealer can extend into the mandibular canal resulting in serious damage to the inferior alveolar nerve. Although there are complex surgical treatments to address this situation, "prevention" is the key word. Initial radiographs can be helpful in determining the proximity of the mandibular canal. Conventional radiographs provide only a two-dimensional image of the relationship between root apex and mandibular canal. CBCT provides vastly more information as a three-dimensional image.

Maxillary Sinus

CBCT radiographs are valuable in determining the relationship between root apices and the floor of the maxillary sinus. Filling material extruded into the sinus has the potential to cause chronic sinusitis and infection. Again, "prevention" is the key word.

7.14 Retreatment Cases

Retreatment cases are usually more challenging than initial root canal therapy. The clinician must often work through crowns or other restorations that complicate access and visibility. In addition, the presence of posts/cores is another issue for the clinician if a nonsurgical approach is dictated by clinical factors. Previous mechanical errors including ledges or perforations may further complicate treatment.

Retreatment cases are particularly prone to exacerbations. Often these cases have had a long history of persistent infection with a complex flora. Microorganisms found in failed endodontically treated teeth either have remained in the root canal following previous treatment or have entered since treatment through coronal leakage. Clinical procedures have the potential to force debris from the canal into the periapical tissues.

It is generally understood that the microbial flora associated with primary root canal infections are polymicrobial and dominated by anaerobes [10]. Secondary root canal infections are composed of fewer species and are dominated by facultative anaerobic Gram-positive bacteria, principally enterococci [14].

A study evaluated postoperative discomfort associated with surgical and nonsurgical endodontic retreatment [11]. They determined that surgical retreatment resulted in more discomfort and tended to bring about greater increased costs than nonsurgical retreatment.

7.14.1 Retreatment Bacterial Flora

An important consideration in retreatment cases is the origin of the intra-canal bacterial flora. The microbial source may be due to a defective restoration or colonies remaining after initial root canal therapy. If the cause of bacterial penetration is the restoration, it must be replaced. Maintaining a defective restoration precludes endodontic success. Microbes remaining after root canal therapy must be addressed as they would in any endodontic case, that is, instrumentation, irrigation, and obturation are the keys to success.

Microbiologically the flora in a failed case is most often less complex than in primary treatment. Cultivation studies demonstrated that the microbiota of persistent or secondary intra-radicular infections associated with endodontic treatment failure, unlike primary infections, is usually composed of only one to two species. Gram-positive facultative bacteria, particularly *Enterococcus faecalis*, are predominant [29]. This virulent microbe is particularly difficult to eliminate due to its resistance to calcium hydroxide, and it can survive without nutrition for long periods of time [25].

The results of that study indicated that *E. faecalis* is significantly more associated with asymptomatic cases of primary endodontic infections than with symptomatic ones. Furthermore, *E. faecalis* was much more likely to be found in cases of failed endodontic therapy than in primary infections [25]. It has been suggested that *E. faecalis* resistance to calcium hydroxide may also be due to a gene involved in cell division which enables it to survive following prolonged exposure to alkaline pH levels [1].

7.15 Persistent Pain Following Seemingly Successful Endodontic Therapy

Some cases with apparently successful endodontic therapy continue to cause pain despite evidence of complete radiographic healing. This outcome is frustrating for the patient and dentist and can result in additional misguided treatment including extraction.

- Studies examined this phenomenon and determined that there are statistically valid predictors that can be useful in identifying such cases prior to initial treatment. A study found the following factors to be of importance as predictors of persistent pain following seemingly successful root canal therapy: presence and duration of preoperative pain from the tooth site, lasting at least 3 months, a positive history of previous chronic pain experience, or painful treatment in the orofacial region and female gender [19, 20, 23].

7.15.1 Frequency of Persistent Pain

A systematic review and meta-analysis also examined the frequency of persistent tooth pain after root canal therapy. It was determined that the frequency of all-cause persistent tooth pain after endodontic procedures was estimated to be 5.3 %, and higher quality studies suggested >7 % [20].

The review determined that there were a number of statistically valid predictors.

Significant predictors of persistent pain:

- Preoperative pain persistent for more than 3 months
- Previous chronic pain problems (4× more likely)
- Inter-appointment pain
- Gender (women 3.8× more likely to develop chronic pain after RCT)
- Preoperative tenderness to percussion [20]

A follow-up study determined that "Non-odontogenic pain is not an uncommon outcome after root canal therapy and may represent half of all cases of persistent tooth pain. These findings have implications for the diagnosis and treatment of painful teeth that were previously root canal treated because therapy directed at the tooth in question would not be expected to resolve non-odontogenic pain" [19].

Possible causes of persistent pain were found to be:

- Untreated canal and failed occlusal seal
- Tooth fracture
- Pain from an adjacent tooth
- Non-odontogenic referred pain
- Deafferentation (the elimination or interruption of afferent nerve impulses)

The predictors of persistent pain, individually and as a group, are useful for the clinician to consider. They may be helpful in identifying cases that may pose postoperative problems. Further research is necessary in this area to understand and validate preoperative findings and their relationship to persistent postoperative pain.

Consideration of a non-odontogenic cause of seemingly endodontic pain is particularly important. It is easy to envision a scenario in which a "painful tooth" is retreated, pain persists, apical surgery is then performed, but pain still persists. An extraction often results but pain may still persist. This unfortunate scenario can result when non-odontogenic causation is not fully considered.

7.16 Self-Assessment

7.16.1 Case 1

A 42-year-old male patient with a noncontributory medical history returns to your office the day after instrumentation, irrigation, and closure of tooth # 3. He complains of severe pain and sensitivity when touching the tooth or masticating. There is no swelling in the muccobuccal fold. Treatment notes indicate that you instrumented three canals to a #20 K file and used rotary instruments. How would you treat this patient?

Answer

- Provide local anesthesia.
- Check occlusion. Reduce occlusion if not already done and restorative considerations permit.
- Confirm measurement.
- If the tooth was instrumented only up to a 20 K file or less, it is likely that tissue was left in the canals.
- Re-instrument all canals to a 25–30 K file and/or rotary instrument.
- Irrigation.
- Place calcium hydroxide dressing.
- Closure.
- Analgesics.

Goal of Treatment

The treatment is biologically based. Confirming the measurement and re-instrumenting should eliminate residual tissue in the canals without further damage to the apical tissues. Occlusal reduction will put the periodontal ligament at rest.

7.16.2 Case 2

A 31-year-old male presents 24 h after endodontic instrumentation. His medical history indicates an allergy to penicillin. He has a large fluctuant swelling in the muccobuccal fold adjacent to #30.

He reports the swelling has increased significantly in the last 12 h, as has his pain. Treatment notes indicate that he presented with an asymptomatic non-vital tooth without a radiolucent lesion. Tooth # 30 was instrumented to a 25 K file and 30 rotary instrument. It was irrigated with sodium hypochlorite. Adjacent teeth have no restorations and no caries. How would you treat this patient?

Answer

- Inferior alveolar nerve block.
- Take the patient's temperature (optional, depending on size of swelling, localization, and presence of malaise).
- Confirm measurement control.
- Re-instrument and enlarge the canals and irrigate with sodium hypochlorite.
- Attempt to establish drainage through the canal.
- Place calcium hydroxide dressing.
- Closure.
- Reduce occlusion, if restorative considerations permit.
- Incision and drainage for the fluctuant swelling.
- Analgesics/antibiotic (note penicillin allergy). Clindamycin is an appropriate substitute.
- Patient should return in 24–48 h for reassessment and re-cleaning/shaping and irrigation.

Goal of Treatment

The suggested approach addresses the microbial cause of the exacerbation. The goal is to eliminate or significantly reduce the intra-canal microbial flora and decompress the periapical tissues.

The use of antibiotics is a supplement to the clinical treatment and is not a "cure" of the basic microbial problem. In a non-vital case (no vascular circulation) little or none of the systemic antibiotic reaches the canal space.

References

1. Appelbe OK, Sedgley CM (2007) Effects of prolonged exposure to alkaline pH on Enterococcus faecalis survival and specific gene transcripts. Oral Microbiol Immunol 22(3):169–174
2. Arias A, De La Macorra JC, Hidalgo JJ et al (2013) Predictive models of pain following root canal treatment: a prospective clinical study. Int Endod J 46(8):784–793
3. Barnett F, Tronstad L (1989) The incidence of flare-ups following endodontic treatment. J Dent Res 68:1253
4. Caviedes-Bucheli J, Azuero-Holguin MM, Correa-Ortiz JA et al (2011) Effect of experimentally induced occlusal trauma on substance p expression in human dental pulp and periodontal ligament. J Endod 37(5):627–630
5. Genet JM, Hart AA, Wesselink PR et al (1987) Preoperative and operative factors associated with pain after the first endodontic visit. Int Endod J 20(2):53–64
6. Hargreaves KM, Cohen S, Berman LH (2011) Cohen's pathways of the pulp. Mosby Elsevier, St. Louis
7. Hasselgren G, Reit C (1989) Emergency pulpotomy: pain relieving effect with and without the use of sedative dressings. J Endod 15(6):254–256

8. Henry M, Reader A, Beck M (2001) Effect of penicillin on postoperative endodontic pain and swelling in symptomatic necrotic teeth. J Endod 27(2):117–123
9. Houck V, Reader A, Beck M et al (2000) Effect of trephination on postoperative pain and swelling in symptomatic necrotic teeth. Oral Surg Oral Med Oral Pathol Oral Radiol Endod 90(4):507–513
10. Kantz WE, Henry CA (1974) Isolation and classification of anaerobic bacteria from intact pulp chambers of non-vital teeth in man. Arch Oral Biol 19(1):91–96
11. Kvist T, Reit C (2000) Postoperative discomfort associated with surgical and nonsurgical endodontic retreatment. Endod Dent Traumatol 16(2):71–74
12. Lin LM, Rosenberg PA, Lin J (2005) Do procedural errors cause endodontic treatment failure? J Am Dent Assoc 136(2):187–193; quiz 231
13. Menezes-Silva R, Khaliq S, Deeley K et al (2012) Genetic susceptibility to periapical disease: conditional contribution of MMP2 and MMP3 genes to the development of periapical lesions and healing response. J Endod 38(5):604–607
14. Molander A, Reit C, Dahlén G et al (1998) Microbiological status of root-filled teeth with apical periodontitis. Int Endod J 31(1):1–7
15. Moos HL, Bramwell JD, Roahen JO (1996) A comparison of pulpectomy alone versus pulpectomy with trephination for the relief of pain. J Endod 22(8):422–425
16. Morsani JM, Aminoshariae A, Han YW et al (2011) Genetic predisposition to persistent apical periodontitis. J Endod 37(4):455–459
17. Nagle D, Reader A, Beck M et al (2000) Effect of systemic penicillin on pain in untreated irreversible pulpitis. Oral Surg Oral Med Oral Pathol Oral Radiol Endod 90(5):636–640
18. Nist E, Reader A, Beck M (2001) Effect of apical trephination on postoperative pain and swelling in symptomatic necrotic teeth. J Endod 27(6):415–420
19. Nixdorf DR, Moana-Filho EJ, Law AS et al (2010) Frequency of nonodontogenic pain after endodontic therapy: a systematic review and meta-analysis. J Endod 36(9):1494–1498
20. Nixdorf DR, Moana-Filho EJ, Law AS et al (2010) Frequency of persistent tooth pain after root canal therapy: a systematic review and meta-analysis. J Endod 36(2):224–230
21. O'keefe EM (1976) Pain in endodontic therapy: preliminary study. J Endod 2(10):315–319
22. Pickenpaugh L, Reader A, Beck M et al (2001) Effect of prophylactic amoxicillin on endodontic flare-up in asymptomatic, necrotic teeth. J Endod 27(1):53–56
23. Polycarpou N, Ng YL, Canavan D et al (2005) Prevalence of persistent pain after endodontic treatment and factors affecting its occurrence in cases with complete radiographic healing. Int Endod J 38(3):169–178
24. Ricucci D, Langeland K (1998) Apical limit of root canal instrumentation and obturation, part 2. A histological study. Int Endod J 31(6):394–409
25. Rocas IN, Siqueira JF Jr, Santos KR (2004) Association of Enterococcus faecalis with different forms of periradicular diseases. J Endod 30(5):315–320
26. Rosenberg PA (2003) Clinical strategies for managing endodontic pain. Endod Top 3:78–92
27. Rosenberg PA, Babick PJ, Schertzer L et al (1998) The effect of occlusal reduction on pain after endodontic instrumentation. J Endod 24(7):492–496
28. Siqueira JF, Barnett F (2004) Interappointment pain: mechanisms, diagnosis, and treatment. Endod Top 7(1):93–109
29. Siqueira JF, Rôças IN (2005) Exploiting molecular methods to explore endodontic infections: part 2–redefining the endodontic microbiota. J Endod 31(7):488–498
30. Siqueira JF, Rôças IN, Provenzano JC et al (2009) Relationship between Fcgamma receptor and interleukin-1 gene polymorphisms and post-treatment apical periodontitis. J Endod 35(9):1186–1192
31. Sjogren U, Hagglund B, Sundqvist G et al (1990) Factors affecting the long-term results of endodontic treatment. J Endod 16(10):498–504
32. Torabinejad M, Kettering JD, McGraw JC et al (1988) Factors associated with endodontic interappointment emergencies of teeth with necrotic pulps. J Endod 14(5):261–266

33. Trope M (1991) Flare-up rate of single-visit endodontics. Int Endod J 24(1):24–26
34. Tsesis I, Faivishevsky V, Fuss Z et al (2008) Flare-ups after endodontic treatment: a meta-analysis of literature. J Endod 34(10):1177–1181
35. Tsuchiya H, Mizogami M, Ueno T et al (2007) Interaction of local anaesthetics with lipid membranes under inflammatory acidic conditions. Inflammopharmacology 15(4):164–170
36. Walton R (2002) Interappointment flare-ups: incidence, related factors, prevention, and management. Endod Top 3:67–76

Therapeutics 8

8.1 Pharmacotherapeutics

8.1.1 Antibiotics

It is important to understand the role of antibiotics in the treatment of endodontic infections. In specific situations, they can play a supportive role in the reestablishment of the proper balance between the host's defenses (immune and inflammatory) and microbes. Clinical and pharmacologic strategies are used independently or in unison to prevent or treat pain and infection.

Antibiotics should be considered as a useful supplement to endodontic cleaning/shaping and irrigation in specific situations. They are not analgesics and should not be used to treat pain. Short-term, high-concentration, broad-spectrum antibiotic prophylaxis is indicated for some heart conditions and in some situations for prosthetic joints [9].

Clinical Tips

- When there are questions concerning antibiotic premedication, it is advisable to communicate with the patient's physician.
- The clinician must stay alert for changes in medical indications for antibiotic prophylaxis as well as dose modifications.

8.1.2 Use and Abuse of Antibiotics

- The American Association of Endodontists, *Colleagues for Excellence*, published a newsletter in 2012, titled "Use and Abuse of Antibiotics." This article reviews the most current guidelines for antibiotic prophylaxis for endocarditis and joint replacement. The newsletter is available at http://www.aae.org/colleagues/.

DOI 10.1007/978-3-642-54701-0_8,

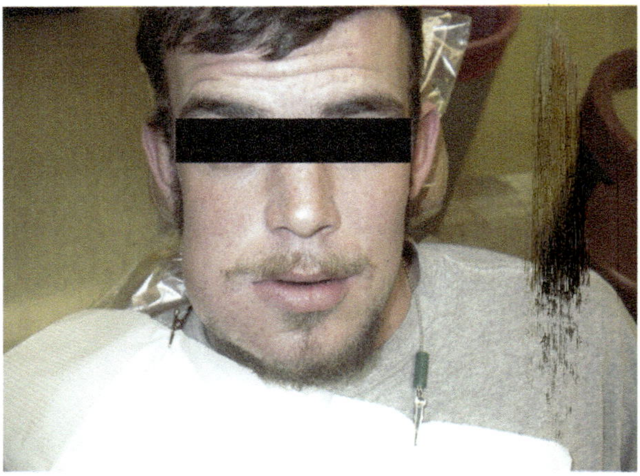

Fig. 8.1 Emergency patient, presenting with cellulitis due to a necrotic mandibular molar

- There are guidelines for the use of antibiotics during endodontic therapy, but each case may present variables that can influence the decision. Not all swellings require antibiotic therapy. For example, a large diffuse swelling increasing in size and producing no drainage on instrumentation may be a candidate for incision and drainage and perhaps an antibiotic. In contrast, a small, well-circumscribed swelling does not usually require antibiotic therapy. Antibiotics may be used in select non-vital cases that meet the criteria described below (Fig. 8.1).

Indications and Contraindications for Antibiotics

The following are important facts concerning the use of antibiotics in the treatment of endodontic infections.

Indications for Adjunctive Antibiotics

- Fever >100 ° F
- Malaise
- Lymphadenopathy
- Trismus
- Increased swelling
- Cellulitis
- Osteomyelitis
- Persistent infection

Conditions Not Requiring Adjunctive Antibiotics

- Pain without signs and symptoms of infection
  - *Symptomatic irreversible pulpitis*
  - *Acute periradicular periodontitis*
- Teeth with necrotic pulps and a radiolucency
- Teeth with a sinus tract (chronic periradicular abscess)
- Localized fluctuant swellings [24]

8.1.3 Facts Concerning the Use of Antibiotics

- The cause of the infection must be addressed (cleaning/shaping and irrigation) prior to, or concomitant with, antibiotic therapy
- Cleaning/shaping and irrigation *without* antibiotic therapy will result in healing of most endodontic infections. The majority of endodontic infections do not require systemic antibiotic therapy.
- It has been estimated that up to 60 % of human infections resolve due to host defenses alone following removal of the cause of the infection without antibiotic intervention.

Antibiotics, Bacterial Susceptibility, and Acute Abscesses

A study examined the susceptibility of bacteria, recovered from acute apical abscesses, to five commonly used antibiotics. Antibiotic susceptibility data drawn from 12 acute apical abscesses led to the following conclusions [2]:

- Pen-V-K is the antibiotic of choice for endodontic infections due to its effectiveness in polymicrobial infections, its relative narrow spectrum of activity against bacteria most commonly found in endodontic infections, and its low toxicity and low cost.
- Clindamycin is the antibiotic of choice for patients allergic to penicillin.
- While amoxicillin and Augmentin (amoxicillin and clavulanic acid) demonstrated higher antibacterial effectiveness than Pen-V-K. Due to the broader antibacterial spectrum of amoxicillin and the increased cost of Augmentin, it was recommended that amoxicillin/Augmentin should be reserved for unresolved infections and patients who are immunocompromised.
- Metronidazole demonstrated the greatest amount of bacterial resistance and is only effective against anaerobes. Therefore, it should not be used alone for the treatment of endodontic infections [2].

Additional Facts Concerning Antibiotics

The following section on the use of antibiotics has been adapted and modified from an excellent publication for the dental community presented by the American Association of Endodontists Colleagues for Excellence, as the winter 2012 edition. It is entitled, "Use and Abuse of Antibiotics" and can be found at www.aae.org/colleagues/.

- Antibiotics that can penetrate into the mammalian cell (erythromycin, tetracycline, clindamycin, and metronidazole) are more likely to affect the host defenses than those that cannot (beta-lactams).
- Tetracyclines may suppress white cell chemotaxis. Most antibiotics (except tetracycline) do not depress phagocytosis.
- The use of multiple antibiotics has not been proven superior to a single antibiotic.
- Bactericidal agents are not always superior to bacteriostatic agents. Bactericidal agents are required for patients with impaired host defenses.

- However, bacteriostatic agents are usually satisfactory when the host's defenses against infections are unimpaired.
- Postantibiotic effects (PAEs—persistent suppression of bacterial growth after previous exposure to antibiotics) are more persistent and reliable with bacteriostatic agents (erythromycin, clindamycin) than with bactericidal agents (beta-lactamase) because the clinical effects of bacteriostatic agents are less dose-dependent.

The following principles of antibiotic dosing have been suggested:

- The shorter the duration of therapy, the lower the risk to the patient for the development of antibiotic-induced toxicity and/or allergy and a reduced risk of developing resistant microorganisms.
- It is advisable to initiate antibiotic therapy with a loading dose (an initial dose higher than the maintenance dose). An antibiotic loading dose should be used whenever the half-life of the drug is longer than 3 h or whenever a delay of 12 h or longer to achieve a therapeutic blood level is expected.
- Most antibiotics used in the treatment of orofacial infections have a half-life shorter than 3 h, but, due to their acute nature, most orofacial infections require therapeutic drug blood levels sooner than 12 h. Steady-state blood levels of any drug are usually achieved in a time equal to three to five times the drug's half-life.
- Amoxicillin has a half-life of one to one-and-a-half hours. A steady-state blood level would then be achieved in three to seven-and-a-half hours thereby leading to a substantial delay in achieving therapeutic antibiotic blood levels. A loading dose of two times the maintenance dose is recommended for acute orofacial infections, which better achieves the goal of rapid, high blood levels rather than initiating therapy with the maintenance dose.
- An oral antibiotic should ideally be administered at dosing intervals of three to four times its serum half-life, particularly if steady-state blood levels are desired (as may be indicated with beta-lactam agents). For example, the serum half-life of Pen-V-K is 0.75 h. Higher continuous blood levels of this antibiotic are more likely to be obtained with 4-h rather than 6-h dosing intervals. The shorter the serum half-life of the drug, the shorter the dosing interval will need to be in order to maintain continuous therapeutic blood levels of the drug.
- A common misconception asserts that prolonged (after clinical remission of the disease) antibiotic therapy is necessary to prevent "rebound" infections from occurring. Orofacial infections do not "rebound" if the source of the infection is eliminated.
- Most orofacial infections persist for 2–7 days and often less. Patients placed on antibiotic therapy for an orofacial infection should be clinically evaluated on a daily basis. When there is sufficient clinical evidence that the patient's host defenses have regained control of the infection and that the infection is resolving or resolved, the antibiotic therapy should be terminated.

Clinical Tips

- When a patient is taking an antibiotic for an endodontic infection, it is essential that the patient be seen frequently for concomitant instrumentation, irrigation, and evaluation.

Bacterial Resistance

Microbial antibiotic resistance is an important issue. Its cause is the use and abuse of antibiotics and a simultaneous decline in research and development of new antimicrobial drugs. In Europe alone, it has been estimated that 25,000 people die every year from antibiotic-resistant bacteria, and that only represents infections that were identified in hospitals.

8.1.4 New American Association for Orthopedic Surgeons/ American Dental Association (AAOS/ADA) Guidelines for Antibiotic Usage

The new AAOS/ADA practice guideline [1] principal recommendation is the following:

> The practitioner might consider discontinuing the practice of routinely prescribing prophylactic antibiotics for patients with hip and knee prosthetic joint implants undergoing dental procedures.

The language of the new recommendation seems somewhat vague. What does "might consider" mean? Also, if we discontinue "routinely prescribing prophylactic antibiotics," what sorts of cases would count as not routine?

Some believe that it is likely that the personal and public health harm of widespread antibiotic use for prophylaxis would outweigh its dubious benefits. It is important for dentists, orthopedic surgeons, and patients to communicate with each other as they decide who should receive prophylaxis and when to discontinue it. The decision concerning antibiotic prophylaxis, at this time, should be made on a case-by-case basis.

8.1.5 Systemic Penicillin and Pain

A prospective, randomized, double-blind study determined that the administration of penicillin did not significantly ($P > .05$) reduce spontaneous pain, pain due to percussion, or the number of analgesic medications taken by patients with untreated irreversible pulpitis [19].

The majority of patients with untreated irreversible pulpitis had significant pain and required analgesics to manage their pain. It was concluded that penicillin should not be prescribed for untreated irreversible pulpitis because penicillin is ineffective for pain relief [19].

8.1.6 Self-Assessment

Question:
A patient presents with acute pain of pulpal origin originating from tooth #30 due to a deep carious lesion. The patient has pain when biting, sensitivity to percussion, and a lingering painful response to cold stimuli. Should an antibiotic be prescribed for this patient?

Answer:
The history and clinical tests indicated that tooth #30 has irreversible pulpitis and extension of the inflammatory process into the periodontal ligament resulting in pericementitis. Proper treatment includes initiating endodontics and prescribing an analgesic. There is no indication for an antibiotic. Due to pericementitis, it would be appropriate to reduce the occlusion.

8.2 Preventive (Preemptive) vs. Reactive Analgesic Strategy

Historically, patients have heard these words, "if you have pain, take the medication." That approach to pain is essentially reactive and does not recognize the biological process resulting in pain.

In that scenario, a clinician waits and, if the patient experiences pain, then reacts. A more biologically based preventive approach relies on our knowledge of tissue damage, mediator release, and the subsequent processes.

Preoperative ibuprofen was shown to delay the onset and decrease the severity of pain. There was an additive effect when it was combined with long-lasting local anesthetic.

The combination provided better pain relief than either one alone [6, 18].

"After acetaminophen (1,000 mg) was administered 30 min prior to surgery, onset of the peak pain was delayed and patient discomfort was decreased 3, 4, and 5 h after surgery."

Clinical Tips

- The use of long-lasting rather than short-acting local anesthetics represents an important part of a pain-preventive strategy by blocking pain impulses from the operative site to higher centers during the immediate postoperative period.

- An additional component of a pain-preventive strategy includes having the patient take analgesics at the treatment visit and later. This strategy is directed at blocking production of mediators associated with pain.
- Analgesics should be taken by the clock rather than when a patient experiences pain.

8.3 Analgesics

Various classes of drugs have been studied for the management of posttreatment endodontic pain [22, 25, 27]. These include nonnarcotic analgesics including NSAIDs, acetaminophens, opioids, and steroids.

Opioids and acetaminophen are considered to act primarily on the central nervous system. In contrast, inflammation-suppressing drugs such as corticosteroids and nonsteroidal anti-inflammatory drugs (NSAIDs) are effective in reducing pain with their action at the site of injury. Combination of NSAIDs with acetaminophen, which apparently acts centrally, is even more effective [14, 15].

Patient's pain perception is complex. Factors include genetics, gender, age, organ function, physiological variables, anxiety, severity and type of pain, social–environmental variables, comorbidities, placebo effect, patient compliance, and pharmacodynamics. However, it is important to remember that the clinical treatment we provide is the key factor.

The effectiveness of treatment for pain depends in part on the strength of the clinician–patient relationship. Pain treatment is never about the intervention alone, but about the clinician and patient working together [23].

8.3.1 Exceptions

Although uncommon, some patients may continue to have pain at moderate to severe levels persisting for days, even after appropriate endodontic intervention. Posttreatment analgesic intervention is required in a significant percentage of endodontic cases.

Numerous clinical studies have evaluated the efficacy of a variety of analgesics for their ability to ameliorate dental pain [5, 6, 14, 15]. Most of these studies have used a third-molar surgical extraction model for evaluation of pain of an acute inflammatory nature. It is important to recognize that there are significant differences between a molar extraction and pain associated with an endodontic problem.

In contrast to an extraction where pain emanates from a socket, endodontic pain is often associated with an inflammatory process within the canal due to incomplete removal of the pulp or from periapical tissues as in pericementitis. The endodontic pain process may be associated with the presence of bacterial by-products, influx of primed immune cells, and activation of the cytokine network and other inflammatory mediators.

When comparing the pain associated with acute postoperative inflammation due to oral surgery, it is possible that the efficacy of analgesics differs from pain associated with the more persistent inflammatory process in endodontic cases.

Other factors may modify a patient's response to an analgesic. Among those factors are a patient's genetics, gender, and level of anxiety. These factors will be reviewed in this chapter.

Clinical Tips

- Some patients presenting with preoperative pain continue to experience pain after endodontic treatment. The pain level can range from mild to severe.
- Moderate to severe postoperative pain rarely lasts more than 24–48 h when the cause has been addressed and analgesics are properly utilized.
- Mild to moderate spontaneous pain is most often well managed by nonsteroidal anti-inflammatory drugs, acetaminophen, or a combination of those drugs.
- Severe pain usually requires the inclusion of an opioid in combination with acetaminophen or an NSAID in order to provide significant relief [10, 17, 18].

8.4 Nonnarcotic Analgesics

8.4.1 Nonsteroidal Anti-inflammatory Analgesics (NSAIDs)

Management of endodontic pain is multifactorial and depends on a combination of endodontic procedures and pharmacotherapy. Nonnarcotic drugs including NSAIDs (e.g., ibuprofen) and acetaminophen and their combination are widely used and highly effective for managing pain of inflammatory origin.

NSAIDs bind to plasma proteins and exhibit increased delivery to inflamed tissue via the extravasation of plasma proteins. These drugs had been thought to produce analgesia through peripheral mechanisms, but the central nervous system is now thought to be an additional site of action.

Ibuprofen is considered the prototype of contemporary NSAIDs and has a well-documented efficacy and safety profile. Other NSAIDs may have some advantages. For example, etodolac (Lodine) has been shown to cause minimal gastrointestinal irritation and ketoprofen (Orudis) has been shown in some studies to be somewhat more analgesic than ibuprofen. A number of NSAIDs have been shown to be more effective analgesics for inflammatory pain than acetaminophen/opioid combinations such as Tylenol no. 3 [10].

8.4.2 Effects of NSAIDs on Pregnant Women and Infants

A cohort study [20] investigated the individual effects of ibuprofen, diclofenac, naproxen, and piroxicam on pregnancy outcome. The main outcome measures were infant survival, congenital malformations, structural heart defects, neonatal complications, hemorrhage during pregnancy and postpartum, and asthma at age of 18 months.

It was determined that one or more of four nonsteroidal anti-inflammatory drugs (NSAIDs) were used by 6,511 pregnant women (7.2 %). No effect on rates of infant survival, congenital malformation, or structural heart defects was found.

Clinical Tips

- The use of ibuprofen in the second trimester was significantly associated with low birth weight [20].

Ibuprofen use in the second and third trimesters was significantly associated with asthma in 18-month-old children. The use of diclofenac in the second trimester was significantly associated with low birth weight, and diclofenac use in the third trimester was significantly associated with maternal vaginal bleeding. No associations with other neonatal complications were found. There was a lack of association with congenital malformations [20].

Important to Note

The significant association between diclofenac and ibuprofen use late in pregnancy and maternal bleeding and asthma in the child, respectively, is consistent with their pharmacologic effects. The increased risk of low birth weight may partly have been caused by underlying inflammatory conditions and was reassuringly similar to the expected baseline risk of low birth weight [20].

Analgesics and Medical Complications

The selection of analgesics may be affected by a patient's medical history. An example of this can be found in a patient with a history of chronic liver disease and or alcoholism (Figs. 8.2 and 8.3).

Clinical Tips

- NSAIDs are contraindicated in patients with ulcers and aspirin hypersensitivity and liver disease [12, 29].

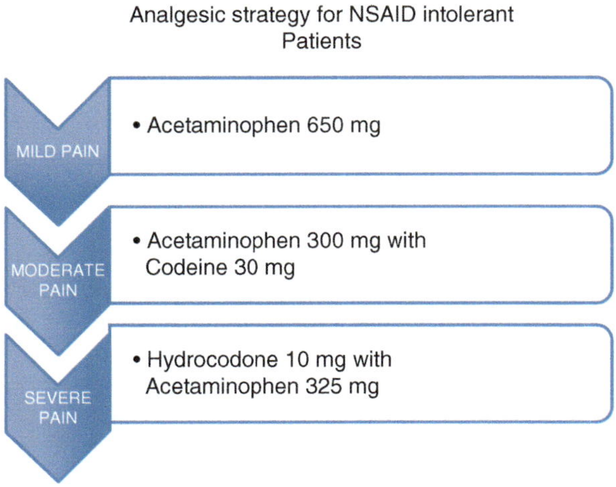

Fig. 8.2 The dose of acetaminophen is under review by the US Food and Drug Administration (FDA). The clinician is advised to review dosage forms of these analgesics as the current recommendations may change

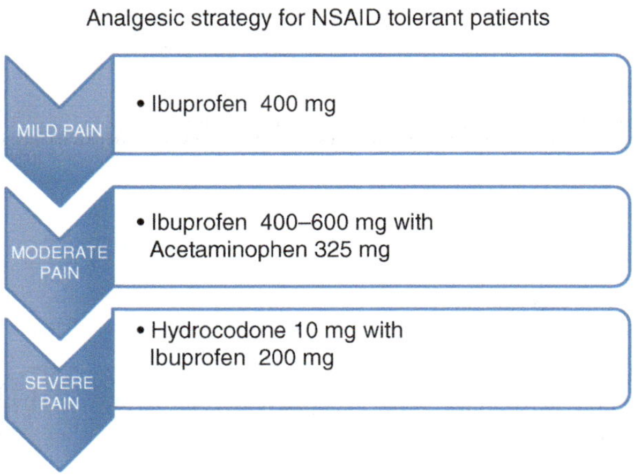

Fig. 8.3 The dose of acetaminophen is under review by the US Food and Drug Administration (FDA). The clinician is advised to review dosage forms of these analgesics as the current recommendations may change

8.5 Acetaminophen (Paracetamol, APAP)

The words "acetaminophen" (used in the United States, Canada, Japan, South Korea, Hong Kong, and Iran) and "paracetamol" used elsewhere originate from para-acetylaminophenol. In some contexts, it is abbreviated as APAP for acetyl-para-aminophenol.

In this text, the words (acetaminophen, paracetamol, and APAP) are used based on the original citation.

8.5.1 Is Acetaminophen Safe?

Although acetaminophen is one of the safest and most effective drugs on the market, it can damage the liver if taken in too high a dose. Acetaminophen overdoses are the number one cause of acute liver failure in the United States.

One cause of inadvertent overdose is that acetaminophen is included in a number of cold remedies and patients may take excessive amounts without realizing it. The appropriate dose of acetaminophen is under review and clinicians are advised to be alert to revisions in the recommended dose.

Important to Note

- Acetaminophen is a widely used analgesic and is commonly found in combination with other drugs for the relief of pain and symptoms of cold or flu.
- The practitioner must be alert to the fact that patients may be taking over-the-counter medications that include acetaminophen and must be factored into the total daily dose of that drug.
- Previously, the healthy adult dose of acetaminophen had been 4 g (4,000 mg) during a 24-h period. The US Food and Drug Administration (FDA) is in the process of revising this dosage downward in an effort to reduce the incidence of liver toxicity.

8.5.2 Acetaminophen: Pregnancy and Children

Pregnant women often take over-the-counter medication. Acetaminophen (APAP, paracetamol) is recommended by physicians to treat fever and pain during pregnancy. Thus, APAP ranks high on the list of medications taken prenatally [26].

However, emerging evidence arising from human trials clearly reveals a significant correlation between APAP use during pregnancy and an increased risk for the development of asthma in children later in life. It has been concluded that further studies are needed to reconsider the safety and dosage of APAP during pregnancy.

There is substantial epidemiological evidence in adults and children that acetaminophen use is associated with asthma symptoms. There is also a considerable body of evidence that supports a modest but consistent association of acetaminophen use during pregnancy and early infancy with asthma in later childhood [11].

There is compelling epidemiological evidence concerning a need to establish guidelines so that appropriate advice and interventions can be developed for pregnant women, mothers, and children at risk of asthma. This requires randomized trials of analgesics and antipyretics, including acetaminophen, in a variety of clinical settings [11].

As noted, there are ambiguous reports concerning increased risk for pregnancy complications such as miscarriage, stillbirth, preterm birth, or fetal malformations upon APAP exposure. APAP can be liver toxic, and since APAP appears to freely cross the placenta, therapeutic and certainly toxic doses could not only affect maternal but also fetal hepatocytes [26, 29].

8.5.3 Opioid Analgesics

Opioids are potent analgesics and are most commonly used in dentistry in combination with acetaminophen, aspirin, and ibuprofen. Most clinically available opioids activate receptors in the brain. Activation inhibits transmission of nociceptive signals from the trigeminal nucleus to higher brain regions, and recent studies indicate that opioids also activate peripheral opioid receptors in the dental pulp [10].

Although opioids are effective as analgesics for moderate to severe pain, their use is limited by their adverse side effects, which can include nausea, emesis, dizziness, drowsiness, and the potential for respiratory depression and constipation. Chronic use is associated with tolerance and dependence. Because dosage is limited by side effects, these medications are almost always used in combination drugs to manage dental pain. A combination formulation is preferred because it permits a lower dose of the opioid, thereby reducing side effects.

It has been reported that the 60 mg dose of codeine (the amount in two tablets of acetaminophen with codeine no. 3) produces significantly more analgesia than placebo, although it often produces less analgesia than either aspirin 650 mg or acetaminophen 600 mg. In general, patients taking only 30 mg of codeine report only about as much analgesia as those taking a placebo. Gender-dependent differences seem to exist in responsiveness to at least the kappa opioid agonists, and women have a significantly greater analgesic response to pentazocine compared to men [10].

Fortunately, non-opioid analgesics are readily available and there is good evidence indicating the effectiveness of combinations of acetaminophen (paracetamol) and ibuprofen.

8.5.4 Recent Research

A powerful clinical study used a double-blind design that was placebo controlled, randomized, and single dose and utilized three sites [5]. The study was designed to compare the efficacy and tolerability of different analgesic combinations, including a novel single-tablet combination of ibuprofen/paracetamol (acetaminophen). It investigated moderate to severe postoperative dental pain following extraction of at least three impacted molars, two of which were mandibular molars [5].

The study compared the following:

- Placebo
- Acetaminophen 500 mg/codeine 15 mg
- Ibuprofen 200 mg/codeine 12.8 mg
- Ibuprofen 200 mg/acetaminophen 500 mg
- Ibuprofen 400 mg/acetaminophen 500 mg

The results were the following:

Ranking of the five treatments (from best to worst)

- Two tablets of ibuprofen 200 mg/acetaminophen 500 mg
- One tablet of ibuprofen 200 mg/acetaminophen 500 mg
- Two tablets of ibuprofen 200 mg/codeine 12.8 mg
- Two tablets of acetaminophen 500 mg/codeine 15 mg
- Placebo

8.5.5 Significance

- This study found that one or two tablets of the single-tablet combination of ibuprofen 200 mg/acetaminophen 500 mg was significantly more effective than two tablets of acetaminophen/codeine or one tablet of the ibuprofen/acetaminophen combination.
- The peak pain relief was found to be higher and more sustained in patients taking two tablets of the single-tablet combination of ibuprofen/acetaminophen (compared with all other treatments.

8.5.6 Adverse Effects

The proportion of subjects reporting adverse effects was statistically significantly less with either one or two tablets of the single-tablet combination of ibuprofen/acetaminophen compared with the codeine analgesic combinations. Codeine is known to be associated with several side effects, including nausea and vomiting [17].

8.5.7 A Recent Critical Analysis

Classic analgesic therapy for the management of acute postoperative pain has relied on orally administered analgesics such as ibuprofen, naproxen and acetaminophen, or *N*-acetyl-*p*-aminophenol (APAP), as well as combination formulations containing opioids such as hydrocodone with APAP.

The combination of ibuprofen and APAP has been advocated as an alternative therapy for postoperative pain management. A critical analysis was conducted in order to evaluate supporting evidence for the use of an ibuprofen–APAP combination after third-molar extractions and propose clinical treatment recommendations for its use in managing acute postoperative pain in dentistry [17].

8.5.8 Results of the Analysis

- Systematic reviews indicated that the ibuprofen–APAP combination may be a more effective analgesic, with fewer untoward effects, than are many of the currently available opioid-containing formulations.

Several randomized controlled trials that also indicated that the ibuprofen–APAP combination provided greater pain relief than did ibuprofen or APAP alone after third-molar extractions [17].

- Adverse effects associated with the combination were similar to those of the individual component drugs.

8.5.9 Clinical Implications

Combining ibuprofen with APAP provides dentists with an additional therapeutic strategy for managing acute postoperative dental pain. This combination has been reported to provide greater analgesia without significantly increasing the adverse effects that often are associated with opioid-containing analgesic combinations.

The strategy of combining two analgesic agents having distinct mechanisms or sites of action, such as combining a peripherally acting analgesic with a centrally acting analgesic, has been advocated for many years. Analgesic formulations containing an opioid and a peripherally acting analgesic consistently provide greater pain relief than do the component agents when administered alone.

An example of a fixed-dose analgesic combination that does not contain an opioid is the formulation of ibuprofen with APAP (Maxigesic) that has been marketed in recent years in New Zealand by AFT Pharmaceuticals (Auckland, New Zealand) [17].

8.6 Addiction to Prescription Analgesics

Addiction to prescription analgesics was originally thought to be a problem associated with men. It was traced back to workers who did labor as coal miners and factory workers in Appalachia. However, a new analysis of data from the United States found that deaths in recent years have been rising far faster among women, quintupling since 1999.

More women now die of overdoses from analgesics like Oxycontin than from cervical cancer. Overdoses in men are increasing according to the data from the US Centers for Disease Control and Prevention. The problem is affecting Caucasian women more than black women and older women more than younger women.

A number of changing societal factors affecting women today may be the cause of this significant problem.

The clinician should be alert for patients who seek medication beyond what is usually required to prevent or control pain. According to a report in the *New York Times*, "Sharp rise in women's deaths from overdose of pain killers," July 2013, prescriptions for analgesics should be limited to what is required to cope with the problem.

8.7 Corticosteroids

Establishing canal patency, instrumenting, and irrigating often cause periapical irritation, resulting in inflammation and pain. Inadvertently, bacteria and canal debris may be pushed into the apical tissues exacerbating the problem. In response to the irritation, inflammatory mediators (e.g., prostaglandins, bradykinin, substance P, etc.) are released into the periapical tissues. As a result, pain fibers are stimulated or sensitized and there is an increase in vascular dilation and permeability. The result is edema and elevated tissue pressure that contributes to patients' pain.

It is well established that glucocorticosteroids can reduce an acute inflammatory response by suppressing vasodilation, migration of polymorphonuclear (PMNs) leukocytes, and phagocytosis and by inhibiting formation of arachidonic acid and its metabolites. This process prevents pain by blocking the COX and lipoxygenase pathways, synthesis of prostaglandins and leukotrienes. Based on this knowledge, researchers have investigated the usefulness of corticosteroids taken either systemically or used in the root canal as a post-instrumentation dressing [13]. The methodologies employed have resulted in varied results and the conclusions drawn from studies are not in agreement and some are contradictory.

8.7.1 Systemic Administration of Steroids (Glucocorticoids) and Postoperative Pain

Steroids have been used to treat endodontic pain because of their potent anti-inflammatory effects [13]. However, they may also have effects on organ systems, but these effects are typically seen only at supraphysiological doses given over a long-term period (usually more than 2 weeks). It has been stated that "a single dose of a glucocorticoid, even a large one, is virtually without harmful effects, and a short course of therapy, up to 1 week, in the absence of specific contraindications, is unlikely to be harmful." This finding was demonstrated in an in vivo study [4]. It was concluded that single large doses (2 mg/kg) of dexamethasone were essentially without harmful side effects. That dose is 10–25 times the amount advocated for endodontic pain relief.

Steroids are contraindicated in patients with systemic fungal infections and known hypersensitivity to the drug. Steroids should be used with caution in patients with ulcerative colitis, pyogenic infection, diverticulitis, peptic ulcer, renal insufficiency, hypertension, osteoporosis, pregnancy, diabetes mellitus, ocular herpes, acute psychosis, and history of tuberculosis. Psychological disturbances have been reported among patients on glucocorticoid therapy. These reactions are reversible and range in severity from mild (euphoria, insomnia, or nervousness) to pronounced (manic–depressive or schizophrenic psychosis). The frequency and severity of adverse effects are correlated to the dose and duration of therapy [28].

Drug interactions associated with the corticosteroids appear to be minimal. There are some drugs that decrease blood levels of the steroid via increased metabolic clearance. These include phenobarbital, phenytoin, rifampin, and ephedrine. Short-term steroid use can produce a reversible suppression of endogenous cortisol production. It has been demonstrated that this suppression is compensated for by adequate amounts of synthetic steroid and therefore prevents manifestations of adrenal insufficiency. NSAIDs should not be used concomitantly with steroids due to increased gastrointestinal adverse effects [28].

Clinical Tips

- Given the relative safety/efficacy relationship between steroids and NSAIDs, most investigators choose an NSAID as the drug of first choice for endodontic postoperative pain control.
- Increasingly, based on recent research (discussed in this chapter), a combination of an NSAID ibuprofen/acetaminophen has gained popularity among clinicians.

8.7.2 Intra-canal Use of Steroids

The most powerful research conclusions are those generated from studies that are prospective, randomized, double-blind, and placebo controlled. None of the endodontic reports on the use of corticosteroids published prior to 1984 meets those criteria, and, therefore, the results should be considered anecdotal.

Results from studies that used corticosteroids in combination with other agents such as an antibiotic and/or an antihistamine are difficult to interpret, as results ascribed to one of the agents may be the result of the combination. Equally difficult to interpret are results from studies using an intra-canal steroid as the means of delivery.

The methodology is critical in those studies and does not account for how much and over what period of time the intra-canal medicament reaches the periapical tissues, the key site of biological activity. Very small concentrations of the agent in question are placed into the canal(s), and apical patency is a factor to consider. To be effective, a quantity (unknown amount) of the medication must pass through the apical foramen due to a concentration gradient against potential back pressure from periapical transudate or exudate. These physical factors were not addressed in the studies thus diminishing their meaningfulness.

8.8 Analgesics and Gender: Research Findings

- Daily use of more than 500 mg of *acetaminophen* increased the risk of high blood pressure by 93 % in older women and by 99 % in younger women.
- Taking more than 400 mg per day of NSAIDs *(ibuprofen, naproxen, and similar drugs)* increased the risk of high blood pressure by 78 % in older women and by 60 % in younger women [8].

8.9 Sex Bias in Research

Male bias has been found to be often present in selecting laboratory animals in biological disciplines [3], and a significant male-orientated bias can also be observed in the preclinical pain literature [16]. Although much more attention has been paid to the topic of sex and/or gender differences in pain in the past few decades [7], there is little evidence to suggest that female mice and rats are becoming more popular as research subjects overall.

The selection of male subjects is associated with their availability and the complication that estrogen levels pose when female subjects are included in studies. Estrogen has anti- and pro-inflammatory components that could complicate the results of studies including females.

It had been assumed that women would respond as men did to analgesics and other drugs. That concept is being increasingly challenged. The omission of female animals from preclinical experiments and females from drug trials can have serious consequences. Failure to appreciate sex differences can lead to either missing biological phenomena entirely or overgeneralization of research findings.

8.9.1 Sex Differences in Response to Opioid Analgesics

In addition to sex differences in pain, differences in the response to opioid analgesics have also been studied. A recent meta-analysis concluded that morphine is moderately more efficacious in women than in men in both clinical (largely patient-controlled analgesia) and experimental studies. However, the picture becomes far less clear for other μ-opioids and especially for mixed μ- and κ-opioid-acting compounds (such as butorphanol, pentazocine, and nalbuphine) [21].

References

1. ADA/AAOS antibiotic prophylaxis guideline for dental patients with orthopedic implants (2013). J Can Dent Assoc 79:d28
2. Baumgartner JC, Xia T (2003) Antibiotic susceptibility of bacteria associated with endodontic abscesses. J Endod 29(1):44–47
3. Beery AK, Zucker I (2011) Sex bias in neuroscience and biomedical research. Neurosci Biobehav Rev 35(3):565–572
4. Czerwinski AW, Czerwinski AB, Whitsett TL et al (1972) Effects of a single, large, intravenous injection of dexamethasone. Clin Pharmacol Ther 13(5):638–642
5. Daniels SE, Goulder MA, Aspley S et al (2011) A randomised, five-parallel-group, placebo-controlled trial comparing the efficacy and tolerability of analgesic combinations including a novel single-tablet combination of ibuprofen/paracetamol for postoperative dental pain. Pain 152(3):632–642
6. Dionne RA (1992) New approaches to preventing and treating postoperative pain. J Am Dent Assoc 123(6):26–34
7. Fillingim RB, King CD, Ribeiro-Dasilva MC et al (2009) Sex, gender, and pain: a review of recent clinical and experimental findings. J Pain 10(5):447–485
8. Forman JP, Rimm EB, Stampfer MJ et al (2005) Folate intake and the risk of incident hypertension among US women. JAMA 293(3):320–329
9. Gutierrez JL, Bagan JV, Bascones A et al (2006) Consensus document on the use of antibiotic prophylaxis in dental surgery and procedures. Med Oral Patol Oral Cir Bucal 11(2):E188–E205
10. Hargreaves KM, Cohen S, Berman LH (2011) Cohen's pathways of the pulp. Mosby Elsevier, St. Louis

11. Henderson AJ, Shaheen SO (2013) Acetaminophen and asthma. Paediatr Respir Rev 14(1): 9–15, quiz 16
12. Little JW, Falace DA, Miller C et al (2012) Dental management of the medically compromised patient. Mosby, St. Louis
13. Marshall JG (2002) Considerations of steroids for endodontic pain. Endod Top 3:41
14. Mehlisch DR, Aspley S, Daniels SE et al (2010) Comparison of the analgesic efficacy of concurrent ibuprofen and paracetamol with ibuprofen or paracetamol alone in the management of moderate to severe acute postoperative dental pain in adolescents and adults: a randomized, double-blind, placebo-controlled, parallel-group, single-dose, two-center, modified factorial study. Clin Ther 32(5):882–895
15. Menhinick KA, Gutmann JL, Regan JD et al (2004) The efficacy of pain control following nonsurgical root canal treatment using ibuprofen or a combination of ibuprofen and acetaminophen in a randomized, double-blind, placebo-controlled study. Int Endod J 37(8):531–541
16. Mogil JS, Chanda ML (2005) The case for the inclusion of female subjects in basic science studies of pain. Pain 117(1–2):1–5
17. Moore PA, Hersh EV (2013) Combining ibuprofen and acetaminophen for acute pain management after third-molar extractions: translating clinical research to dental practice. J Am Dent Assoc 144(8):898–908
18. Moore PA, Werther JR, Seldin EB et al (1986) Analgesic regimens for third molar surgery: pharmacologic and behavioral considerations. J Am Dent Assoc 113(5):739–744
19. Nagle D, Reader A, Beck M et al (2000) Effect of systemic penicillin on pain in untreated irreversible pulpitis. Oral Surg Oral Med Oral Pathol Oral Radiol Endod 90(5):636–640
20. Nezvalova-Henriksen K, Spigset O, Nordeng H (2013) Effects of ibuprofen, diclofenac, naproxen, and piroxicam on the course of pregnancy and pregnancy outcome: a prospective cohort study. BJOG 120(8):948–959
21. Niesters M, Dahan A, Kest B et al (2010) Do sex differences exist in opioid analgesia? A systematic review and meta-analysis of human experimental and clinical studies. Pain 151(1):61–68
22. Okeson JP, Falace DA (1997) Nonodontogenic toothache. Dent Clin North Am 41(2): 367–383
23. Pizzo PA, Clark NM (2012) Alleviating suffering 101–pain relief in the United States. N Engl J Med 366(3):197–199
24. Reader A, Nusstein J, Drum M (2011) Successful local anesthesia for restorative dentistry and endodontics. Quintessence, Chicago
25. Riley JL, Gilbert GH (2001) Orofacial pain symptoms: an interaction between age and sex. Pain 90(3):245–256
26. Thiele K, Kessler T, Arck P et al (2013) Acetaminophen and pregnancy: short- and long-term consequences for mother and child. J Reprod Immunol 97(1):128–139
27. Wall PD, McMahon SB, Koltzenburg M (2006) Wall and Melzack's textbook of pain. Elsevier/ Churchill Livingstone, Philadelphia
28. Williamson LW, Lorson EL, Osbon DB (1980) Hypothalamic-pituitary-adrenal suppression after short-term dexamethasone therapy for oral surgical procedures. J Oral Surg 38(1):20–28
29. Wynn RL, Meiller TF, Crossley HL (2012) Drug information handbook for dentistry: including oral medicine for medically compromised patients & specific oral conditions. Lexi Comp, Hudson

Afterword

When I initiated this project, my goal was to share everything I have learned about endodontic pain with other clinicians. I have learned from so many different sources over many, many years. I have benefitted from the dental and non-dental literature, countless lecturers, faculty, students, and patients. Each patient presents their own challenges, and the information presented in this text may have to be modified in order to meet the specific needs of a patient.

It is my hope that you have found the information in this text to be meaningful. As stated at the outset, pain-free endodontics is a realistic goal. Relieving a patient of severe pain is a uniquely satisfying experience. It is wonderful to see a patient smile at the conclusion of treatment and state something like, "I had heard such terrible stories about root canal treatment, but this was really nothing to be afraid of."

Best wishes and good luck in your future endodontic endeavors.

Paul A. Rosenberg

P.A. Rosenberg, *Endodontic Pain*,
DOI 10.1007/978-3-642-54701-0, © Springer-Verlag Berlin Heidelberg 2014

Index

P.A. Rosenberg, *Endodontic Pain*,
DOI 10.1007/978-3-642-54701-0, © Springer-Verlag Berlin Heidelberg 2014

GPSR Compliance

The European Union's (EU) General Product Safety Regulation (GPSR) is a set of rules that requires consumer products to be safe and our obligations to ensure this.

If you have any concerns about our products, you can contact us on ProductSafety@springernature.com

In case Publisher is established outside the EU, the EU authorized representative is:

Springer Nature Customer Service Center GmbH
Europaplatz 3
69115 Heidelberg, Germany

Batch number: 10584666

Printed by Printforce, the Netherlands